tao paths
good fortune

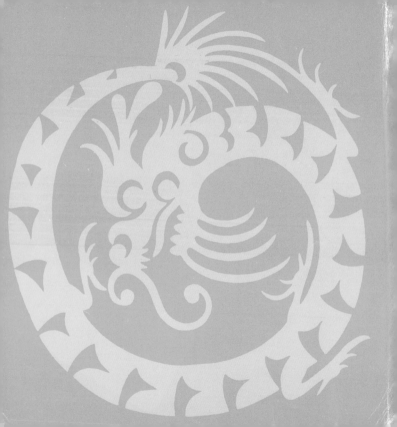

tao paths

good fortune

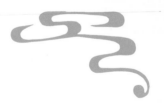

Andrews McMeel
Publishing

Kansas City

Contents

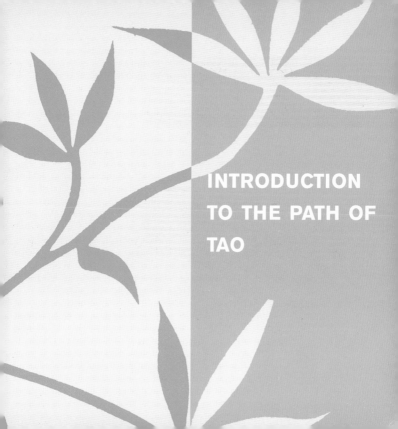

INTRODUCTION
TO THE PATH OF
TAO

We are all born with some good fortune. This comes from a combination of factors that include past-life influence; the physical, emotional, and spiritual health of our parents at the moment of our conception; our early childhood experiences; our environment; our astrological makeup; our own constitutional structure (*jing*); and lastly, our ability to deal with challenges, both internal and external.

The Taoist attitude toward good fortune is based on concepts of fate, destiny, karma (a Buddhist term), and self-cultivation. All of these factors need to be taken into consideration. It is in how we use our unique gifts to work with our particular challenges that enables spiritual cultivation and advancement.

In other words we are, in many ways, masters of our own fate. While it is certainly true that we are all given various and different challenges in this life, we are also given various and different gifts that will help us rise to those challenges.

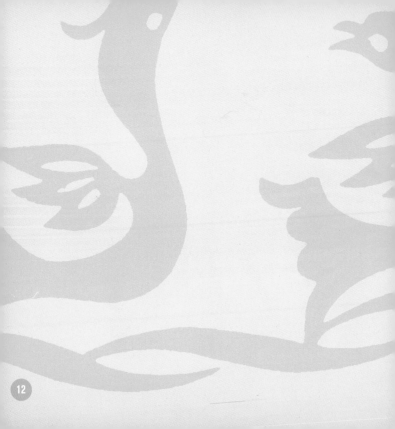

The Path of Tao is one of wholeness, balance, and harmony. It began eight thousand years ago in China, yet continues today wherever anyone follows these basic principles. It is less a religion and more a philosophy. It is a way to work with change rather than against it.

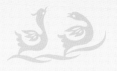

The Path of Tao is a Path of least resistance, of going with the flow of Nature (*wu wei*). It uses the metaphor of water, which adapts itself to the shape of whatever container it finds itself in, always flowing to the low places and, though soft and yielding, can, over time, cut its way through solid rock.

Lao Tzu, the great ancient sage of Tao, said that the Path of Tao is one of seeing simplicity in the complicated and achieving greatness in small things. It is a Path that respects and even honors the Value of Worthlessness and the Wisdom of Foolishness.

Chuang Tzu, the other great sage of Tao, says, "Those who follow the Tao are strong in body, clear of mind, and sharp of sight and hearing. They do not fill their mind with anxieties and are flexible in adjusting to external conditions."

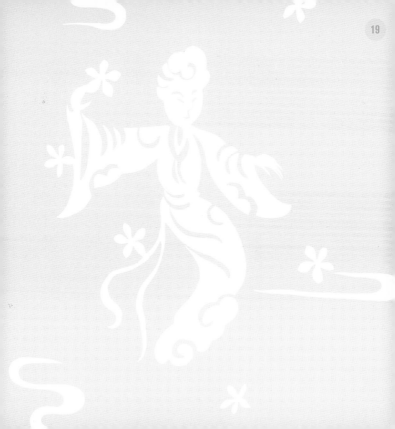

The Path of Tao is a way of life followed by the peasant, the farmer, the gentleman philosopher, and the artist. It is a way of deep reflection and learning from Nature, which is considered to be the highest teacher.

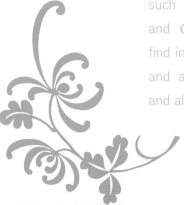

The Path of Tao offers us a simple, practical way of being and living, a way of comforting ourselves on our journey between birth and death and beyond. In wonderfully illustrative texts such as the *Tao Te Ching* and *Chuang Tzu*, we can find inspiration, illumination, and advice on life, death, and all that lies between.

In Chinese medicine practices, we can find cure and comfort for many modern and not-so-modern ills and complaints. The practices of *chi kung* and *tai chi* can give us ways to stabilize and balance our bodies, allowing us to lead long-lasting and healthy lives. Taoist advice on sexuality and relationship can guide us gracefully through the difficult labyrinth of human sexuality.

And through Taoist spiritual and meditation practices we may finally arrive at that precious point of power described in the Taoist tradition as Returning to the One—the source of our own being as well as being-ness itself.

The *Tao Paths* series offers quotes from the traditional Taoist works as well as jewels of wisdom from contemporary Taoist masters. Alongside these words of wisdom you will find stories to delight, mystify, and enlighten you to the deep layers of Taoist thought and practice.

Covering a wide range of Taoist tradition, the books in the *Tao Paths* series explore the ways in which the ancient sages as well as the modern masters have given us tools and practices to plumb the depths of our being and reunite us with our eternal source, the Tao itself.

Tao Paths, Love teaches how to maintain healthy relationships—emotionally, psychologically, and sexually—and how to study the relationship between ourselves and the natural world around us and the infinite depth of our own internal world.

Tao Paths, Harmony teaches how to be at one with the world around us.

Tao Paths, Long Life teaches not only how to achieve a long and healthy life but how to live fully in each moment.

Tao Paths, Good Fortune explores the realms of destiny, karma, and good fortune.

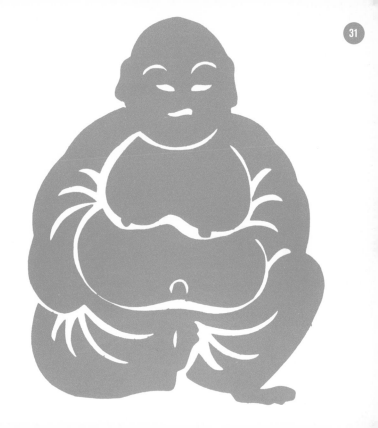

The problems of today are real, profound, often seem unresolvable, and call for something that can be applied to everyday life. The Path of Tao offers not a way out, but a way through. Its advice and wisdom is real and eminently applicable, regardless of race, religion, or gender.

What the men and women of Tao learned in ancient times, through countless years of observation and practice, can be just as useful today as it was in the era of the legendary Yellow Emperor.

Remember that the Path of Tao is not just an ancient, foreign, mystical path; it is a cross-cultural, non-sexist, practical, even scientific way of viewing the world and our place within it. It's practices and philosophy work on many different levels—physical, emotional, psychological, and spiritual.

41

The roots of Tao go back thousands of years; the knowledge gleaned over the centuries can be as helpful for the modern world as in the Tang Dynasty. It can guide us onto the path of least resistance, help us find a way to work with the currents of change and renewal, and allow us to feel a sense of connection to the sacred.

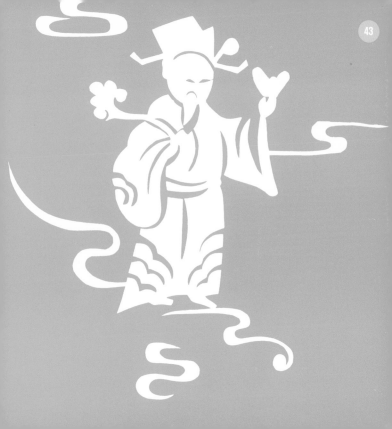

You will meet many strange and wonderful characters in these pages—from the lofty wisdom of Lao Tzu to the often ridiculous metaphors of Chuang Tzu to the down-to-earth tales of Lieh Tzu.

In between, you will meet hunchbacks, cripples, lords and servants, wise sages, and foolish seekers after Truth. But pay attention, you may meet yourself here.

Good fortune can mean prosperity, good health, happiness, mental clarity, emotional balance, or spiritual fulfillment. We each have our own idea and experience of good fortune. And we must each work, in our own way and in our own time, to find our sense of good fortune. In this way, we shall be able to claim it as our own, in this life and into the next.

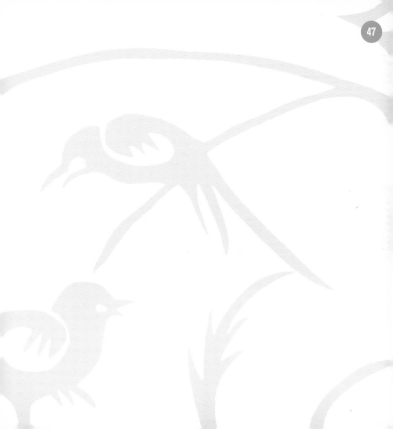

Good fortune can be seen as a gift, a birthright, a goal, a practice, a dream, or a "work in progress." We can use the tools of virtue, grace, right timing, right placement, and spiritual practice, in all its many and varied aspects, to achieve this.

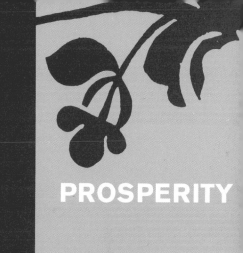

PROSPERITY

Prosperity has always been of concern to most people, never more so than in ancient China. While strict Taoists might have scorned worldly wealth, most people who followed the Way as householders were concerned with prosperity or the lack of it. And while social status was strictly controlled in Chinese society, people did what they could to increase their prosperity and show themselves off at whatever level they could afford.

53

In seventh century B.C.E the *Guanzi* recommended that restrictions be placed on food, clothing, housing, domestic animals, attendants, boats, carriages, and utensils—all according to status. Not only that but there were restrictions regarding hats, clothing, salaries, land, houses, and even after death on coffins, funerals clothing, and graves.

Ancient Chinese society was fluid, and people could rise above their natural station in life, for example, by passing the Imperial examinations. Indeed, scholars were considered to be at the pinnacle of society and when appointed, improved the status of their whole family and often their whole village.

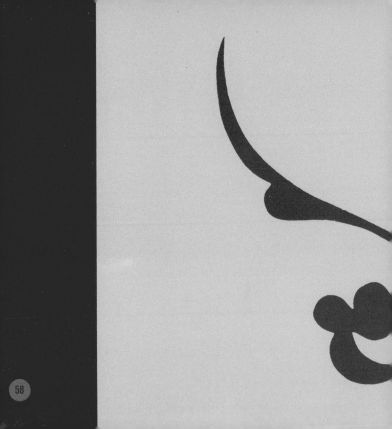

58

The Chinese are great believers in using the spiritual world to help with the pursuit of good fortune and prosperity. The use of talismans, charms, prayers and invocations, and a lot of good old hard work were all employed in the pursuit of prosperity. Also included was the ability to "eat bitter" (*bi ku*), or be able to withstand a great amount of suffering to get to where you wanted to go.

In today's ever-shifting economy, people are no less interested in the pursuit of prosperity. The Path of Tao provides us with ways and means that we can apply to our own situation.

Prosperity is relative. What may seem like riches to one person will seem like poverty to another. How do we know when we have enough? What is enough?

Not singling out certain people for honors

Will stop people from quarreling.

Not collecting riches

Will prevent people from stealing.

By not desiring too many things

Your heart will not be in disorder.

LAO TZU

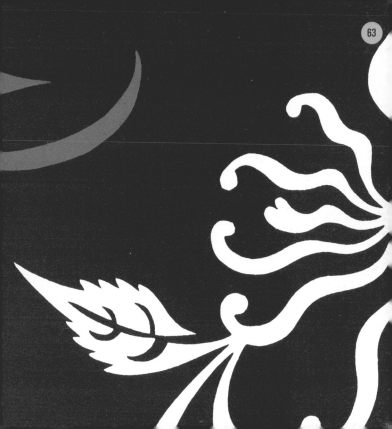

There was once a poor man who begged every day in the center of the marketplace. He was there for so long that people got tired of seeing him there, day after day, and so stopped giving him anything.

So he went to the stables of the T'ien family and got a position as assistant to the horse-doctor there. His old friends made fun of him, saying, "Don't you think it's disgraceful to be the assistant of the horse doctor?"

"To me there is nothing more disgraceful than having to beg for a living," he answered them. "If I was not disgraced by being a beggar, how can I be disgraced by being the assistant to a horse doctor?"

LIEH TZU

Pride can be a very destructive force. By always wanting to be better or higher or richer or more famous than they are, many people never find happiness.

Chinese culture is rich with symbols and word links. The use of calligraphy and pictographs exist not only as works of art but there is believed to be inherent power in them to effect changes in one's financial and social condition.

Life in Chinese villages is often harsh and often dreary, yet generally the future is faced optimistically, even though tinged with a generous amount of fatalism.

RONALD G. KNAPP

The ever-changing cycles of the seasons, the unfolding of year upon year, all give us the opportunity to invoke the spirit of prosperity in many different ways.

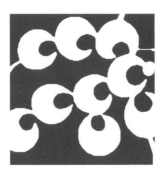

The Chinese word for happiness,
good fortune, blessing, or
luck is *fu*. It also signifies the
idea of bestowal or
receipt of divine favors.

Fu is the intangible power which brings advantage to humankind.

RONALD G. KNAPP

The beauty of the Path of Tao is that there is nothing to join, no vows to take, no special naming or clothing style to follow, no reason to give up your own religion or culture to benefit from its wisdom. Its teachings can be applied on many different levels, in many different circumstances.

Today, in China, there are temples of Taoism, a religious form of Tao (*tao jio*), complete with priests, liturgy, and rituals. But the original philosophical form of Taoism (*tao jia*) was intended as a way of life. It is this form of Taoism that we will be working with.

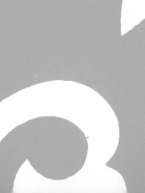

A homonym of *fu*, and an image that is thought to invoke blessings and good fortune, is the bat.

 While the bat is usually thought of in a negative fashion in the West, in China it is a symbol of wealth and good fortune, often seen on walls, paintings, and even ceilings.

There once lived a man in Ch'i who was obsessed with gold. One day he got up at dawn; he got dressed and set out for the marketplace. He went over to the stall that dealt in gold, snatched up a great gold bar and ran off down the street. He was apprehended by the police, who asked him, "What did you think you were doing stealing someone else's gold right in front of so many people?"

"When I took the gold," he replied, "I did not see any other people, I only saw the gold."

LIEH TZU

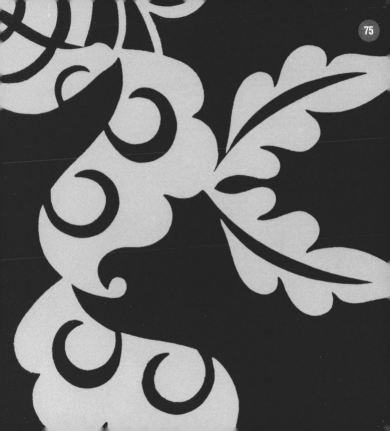

Many times we are so caught up in the pursuit of wealth that we do not have time for anything else. Prosperity is fine, but to lose sight of what is truly valuable in life is to become deluded and blind like the man of Ch'i.

There are five ways that good fortune or happiness can be depicted: longevity (*shou*), wealth (*fu*), health (*kangning*), love of virtue (*youhaode*), and to die a natural death in old age (*kaozhongming*).

Associated with *fu* is the color red or vermilion. Red is the color of summer, the time of expansion and joy. At the New Year, the character for *fu* is written with black or gold ink on red paper. It is pasted outside the doors or gates of many homes in China in order to invoke the spirit of good fortune and prosperity for the coming year.

Poetic couplets are often hung above or alongside doorways or on walls in order to inspire the inhabitants of the home. Some examples include:

"The five blessings have arrived at the door," "The star of good fortune shines brightly on this working household," "The joyous vapors reside eternally with this fortunate family."

A common symbol is that of "double happiness," formed by joining together two characters for joy. Cut from red paper, these are found on walls, doors, and furniture all over China.

The character *shou*, for longevity, is often pictured with four bats (*fu*) encircling it as a symbol of a long life of happiness and prosperity.

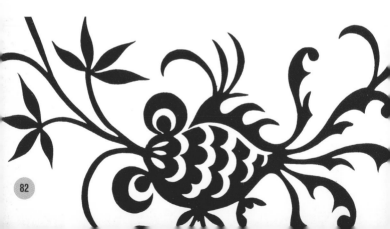

The struggle to pass examinations and achieve financial advantage is epitomized by the carp, a fish that must battle the currents to reach Longmen, the Dragon Gate.

RONALD G. KNAPP

The fish itself is also a symbol of wealth, especially the goldfish, since the character for goldfish, *jin yu*, sounds like "gold in abundance." When pictured alongside a lotus flower, the goldfish evokes "gold and jade joined together" (*jin yu tonghe*), because the word for jade is also *yu*.

Flowers such as red peonies and hibiscus are usually seen as symbols of wealth and prosperity. Also found on many carvings is the plum blossom, its five petals a symbol of the "five good fortunes."

Paintings such as that of the Taoist immortal Shou Xing, the god of immortality, are often shown with the characters for "good fortune," "riches," "longevity," and "joy." He is usually pictured as an old man with a gigantic forehead, a long white beard, a staff of gnarled wood, and holding a gigantic peach of immortality. Many carvings or paintings of this Taoist immortal and symbol of longevity and good fortune are given as birthday gifts.

Po Yi was a poor man who tried to live such a pure life that he eventually starved himself to death. Other, wealthier men, push themselves so hard to acquire yet more wealth that they injure their health and die an early death. Because of this, it could be said that poverty and wealth are both injurious to one's life. What, then, is the correct way to live?

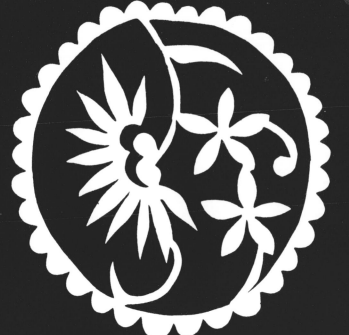

If we have too much wealth we will worry about losing it. If we are too poor, we will be too busy trying to stay alive to enjoy our life. Our basic needs in life need to be met: food, shelter, warm clothing. Also of great importance is enough free time to enjoy other pursuits. Once we have enough for our needs in life, it is time to stop. The endless pursuit of more wealth will kill us just as easily as poverty will.

LIEH TZU

We are all unique in our needs and wants once we rise above substance level. Some people like to travel, some like to collect art, some like to store their riches in a vault. It is the quest for riches that can be our undoing, especially if we do not pay attention to the details of our lives as we go along.

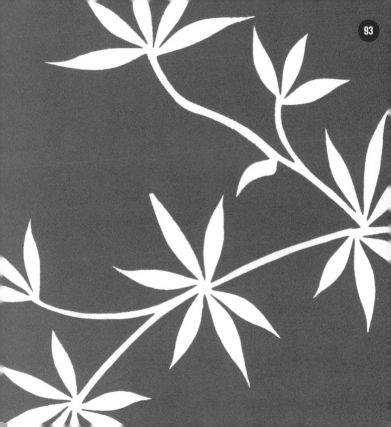

Peace is easy to maintain;

Things are easier to plan for before they happen;

The fragile is easily broken;

The small is easily scattered.

Take action before things happen;

Set things in order before there is disorder.

A great tree is born from a tiny seed;

A great tower is built from a basket of earth.

The journey of a thousand miles begins with
your first step.

LAO TZU

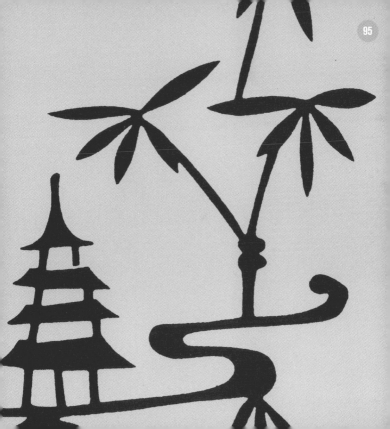

Self-confidence has been quoted as being one of the most important steps to prosperity. This is different from being deceitful. Self-confidence is, instead, the ability to believe in yourself and to be able to pass that belief on to others that you come into contact with.

It is often said that those who are least attached to being prosperous are more likely to achieve it. Those who worry, obsess, and drive themselves relentlessly, will, even if they achieve prosperity, be too tired to enjoy it!

Tuan-mu Shu had inherited his family fortune, said to be worth ten thousand pieces of gold. He never had to work and lived in a fabulous mansion, surrounded with gardens, lakes, terraces, and pavilions. His food and clothing, as well as that of his various wives and concubines, were of the finest quality. He went wherever he wished, traveling far and wide, collecting treasures and exploring anything that he became interested in.

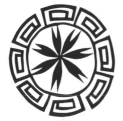

 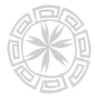 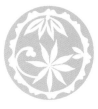 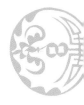

Every day he had hundreds of guests, and it was said that the fires in his kitchen were never allowed to go out; he and his guests were entertained by the finest musicians and dancers in the land. The leftovers of his banquets were distributed far and wide and his generosity for anyone in need was legendary.

Then, when he reached the age of sixty, he suddenly changed his life completely. He gave away all of his wealth and possessions, not even saving some for his wives and children. Finally, he became ill and was too poor to pay for a doctor and so died.

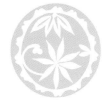

His children had no money to pay for a funeral, but the townspeople, remembering his generosity to them over the years, took up a collection. This was more than enough to pay for his funeral, with enough left over to give to his family.

A prominent Confucian heard about this and he called Tuan-mu Shu a madman, and said he had disgraced his ancestors.

When the Taoist master heard about it he laughed and called him enlightened. "This man was in touch with his essential self," he said, "he lived by his own spirit and never did anything that went against his true nature."

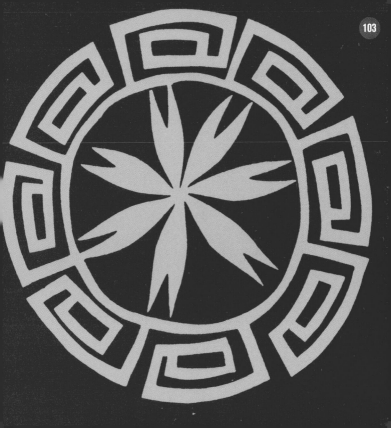

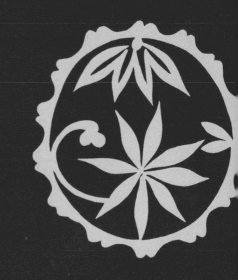

He spent his money when he had it and then gave it away when he no longer needed it. Some may say he was crazy for abandoning his wealth and even the wealth of his family but all he did was follow his own heart, without any constraints or worries about the future. His mind was of such a subtle nature that most people could never understand him.

LIEH TZU

It is said, "You can't take it with you."
This means that, no matter how much
wealth we build up in life, at death, we
must leave it all behind.

Wealth can be measured in different ways. Love, respect, memories, sharing with others, learning new things, going to new places—all of these can be thought of as wealth.

Real wealth cannot be taken away from you. It cannot be lost. It cannot be stolen. It cannot be forgotten.

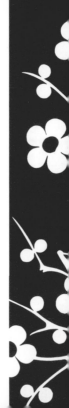

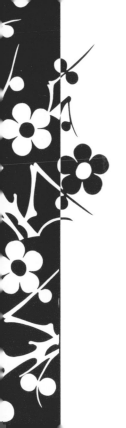

Wealth is valued for
what can be attained
and accomplished by
the means it affords.
One who only hoards
wealth and does not
put it to good use
cannot obtain the full
benefit of wealth.

THOMAS CLEARY

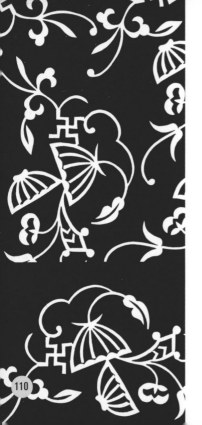

The ability to work with others is very important for any kind of success. When we band together in common interest, we can accomplish much more than any of us can do alone.

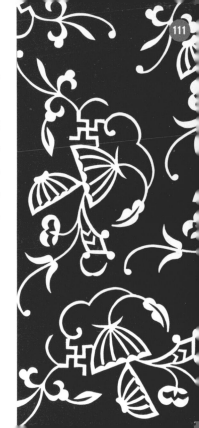

In olden times, people were satisfied with much less than today. We must not be fooled by the advertising that tries to convince us that they know what we need better than we ourselves do.

Spirituality and prosperity can exist together. It is not more spiritual or moral to be poor. If we achieve our success in a virtuous fashion, then we deserve it.

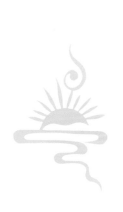

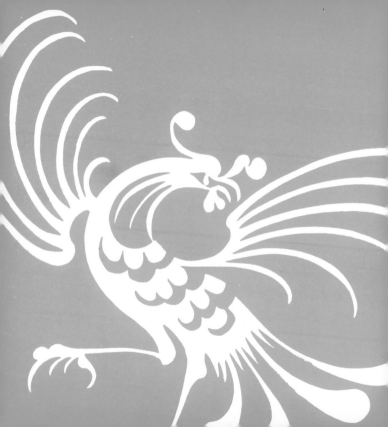

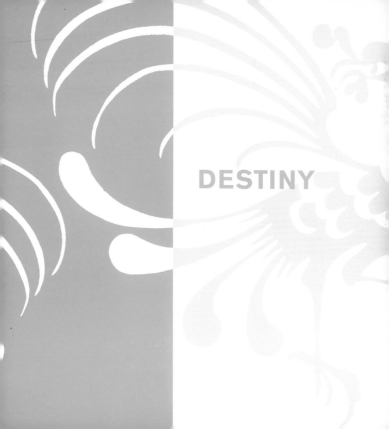

DESTINY

The Chinese word for destiny is *tien ming*, "the decree of Heaven." In ancient times it was thought that destiny or fate was something that was bestowed from Heaven. The Chinese word for heaven, *ti*, describes a sort of celestial mandate. Chinese thought, and Taoism in particular, does not subscribe to the belief in a personal godhead who judges and punishes or rewards.

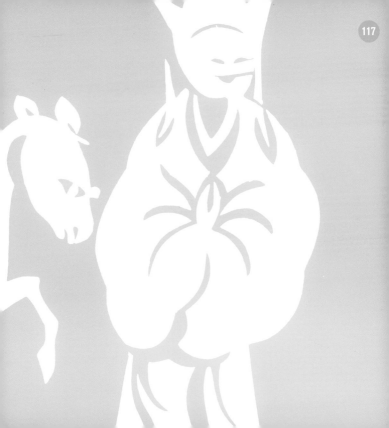

What is called karma is that universal law "you shall reap what you sow." In other words, instead of a great judge in the heavens meting out punishments and rewards, it is our very actions that set up the dynamics of whether we suffer or are rewarded.

There are profound lessons involved here, things that we learn over a lifetime or more. It is believed by the Taoists that spiritual cultivation not only clears any bad karma we have accrued, both in this lifetime and others, but will create new, positive karma that continues after our death.

While there is certainly order and balance in the Tao, there is also a certain amount of random chaos. It is when we get caught up in that chaotic state of things that we often feel oppressed or victimized.

Life consists of many kinds of steps. Sometimes we seem to go forward, at other times we seem to go backward. Sometimes the steps are smooth and clear, other times they are bumpy and uncertain.

If we pay close attention to what is happening and try to find the reality of the situation, we can then respond naturally to it. In this way we will not only be dealing with the situation in a self-aware state but will be creating new, positive karma at the same time.

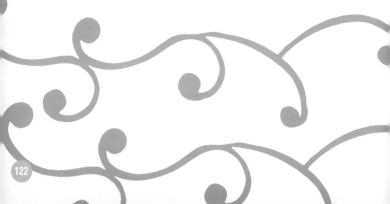

In order to attain a state of getting where there is no past to weigh upon the present and no future to be determined, followers of Tao must reach a profound merging with Tao.

DENG MING DAO

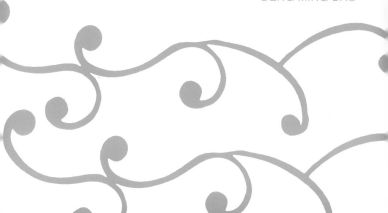

On the Path of Tao we believe that the only constant is change. No matter what the situation is, sooner or later it will change. Of course this is good news when things are bad but not so welcome when our life is good and we would like it to stay that way.

Just as we need to keep in mind that a bad situation will eventually change into something else, we cannot be assured that it will necessarily be a positive change. We must be willing to make the kind of changes in our own being that will allow that situation to evolve into a positive and harmonious one.

Often it is our very own efforts to improve ourselves and our situation in life that impedes that very progress. If our approach is too heavy-handed, if we are too attached to the outcome, if we lose track of the essential things of life in our quest for success and prosperity, we will lose our sense of natural self and consequently suffer for it.

We often become attached to things, situations, or even people that were helpful and appropriate to one part of our life. But if we are interested in growing and progressing in life, we sometimes have to leave those things behind. While it is important to do it in a graceful and compassionate way, we need to give ourselves permission to change and grow in our life.

You need a raft to cross a
river. But once you cross,
you no longer need the raft.
You need to learn the rules
to learn how to do
something. But once you
have learned it you can
forget the rules.

HUANG YUAN CHI

Some people seem to get all the breaks. They are born with strong, healthy bodies, they are charming, personable, intelligent, and even physically attractive. Because of this, people respond to them positively and it seems they do not have to work as hard as the others to get what they want.

The ancient sages were called sages because when they did good deeds or helped people out of difficult situations they did not stay around to be congratulated and adulated but instead often disappeared. This is called "retiring when your work is done."

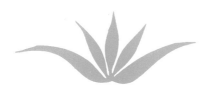

The highest sage shares his moral
possessions with others.
The next in wisdom shares his material
possessions with others.
The man who because of his own
wisdom looks down on others
has never won men's hearts.
The man who in spite of his own
wisdom is humble to others
has never failed to win men's hearts.

LIEH TZU

While it is always good to help others in the physical world, it can be equally helpful to offer emotional or spiritual support. Food and shelter are essential, but there is more to life than survival. Often what people are really looking for in life is what is intangible yet very real and lasting.

What may seem an unfortunate turn of events now will prove to be a blessing in the long run. Likewise, what may now seem to be a fortunate event may prove, in the long run, to be an unfortunate one.

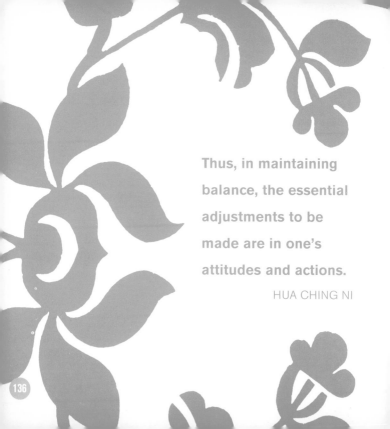

Thus, in maintaining balance, the essential adjustments to be made are in one's attitudes and actions.

HUA CHING NI

It is often our internal approach to a problem or situation that is even more important than whatever outer form our actions may take. It is also on the internal planes that we have the most control and influence, both on the situation itself and our own personal well-being.

If we have no power to change the past and cannot, as yet, have any power over the future, then the present moment is where we need to focus our energies and intent.

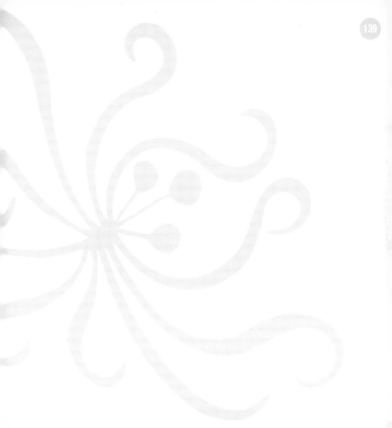

The ancient masters have taught us that joy often follows suffering, that sometimes joy is even given birth from our suffering. If we learn to deal with the inevitable suffering with grace, patience, and insight, we can turn that suffering into a kind of joy.

It is not required that we learn to enjoy our suffering, or that we become some sort of masochistic martyr. What we are talking about here is a kind of active acceptance of suffering as a natural, unavoidable part of life.

The ancient masters
were subtle and profound.
They were so deep they
cannot be known.
Since they cannot be known,
We must try to describe them.

> They were cautious, like someone
> crossing a river in winter.
> They were vigilant, like someone
> surrounded by enemies.
> They were dignified, like honored
> guests.
> They were ephemeral, like melting ice.

They were simple, like an uncarved block of wood.
They were open, like a valley.
They were deep, like swirling water.

LAO TZU

In listing the attributes of the ancient masters, Lao Tzu is giving us a sort of map of how we can conduct ourselves in this confusing, chaotic, and often challenging world.

Often, when we feel stuck and powerless about our situation, if, instead of racking our brains for a solution to change things, we simply stop and wait; things have a way of sorting themselves out.

It takes patience and a special sort of courage to sit and breathe our way through a difficult time. But it can be done.

By practicing the Taoist principles of *wu wei* (not doing anything against the natural flow), of *pu* (being simple like an uncarved block of wood), being like water (which takes whatever shape it's put in and flows downhill to the lowest places), and above all, the patience to sit and breathe and allow things to unfold in their own time, we can become like those ancient masters.

Those who can keep to the Way fit in without making a show and stay forever hidden. Hence they don't leave any tracks.

WANG CHEN

The time we live in now is also a time of sages and masters. In many ways, they are needed now more than ever before. But they are often humble and even invisible.

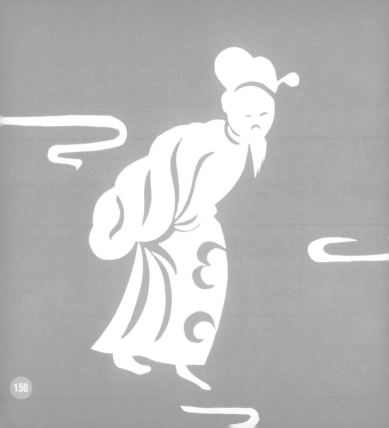

We are cocreators of our own reality. While some seem to be destined to act on the world stage and influence many people, others are working in a very limited yet vital way to raise healthy children, maintain a strong marriage bond, or even be of crucial assistance to a few people.

Yang Pu came to his older brother Yang Chu and asked him, "Suppose there are two men who are equal in age, intelligence, appearance, and talent. But while one man is rich the other is poor.

152

One of them has a long life while the other dies a young man. One man is loved and respected by everyone around him while the other man is despised. Why is it that one enjoys the favors of heaven while the other does not, when they both start out the same way?"

"The ancient ones had a saying," answered Yang Chu. "Everything that happens without our understanding is called destiny. Everything that happens for obscure or confusing reasons is also called destiny.

Now for the one who trusts in destiny there will be no difference between a long life or a short one. If you understand the natural order of things there will be nothing in life to either approve or reject. If you trust in yourself you will not need to fear danger. If you are true to your essential nature you will not be moved by outside forces."

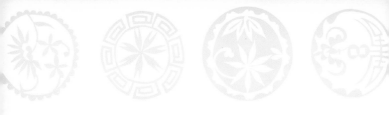

Trusting in the natural unfolding of things, she can go where she pleases and do what needs to be done. The opinions and actions of others will have no effect on her.

LIEH TZU

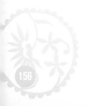
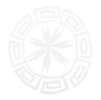
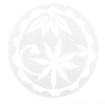

Destiny only has the power that we ourselves give it. We all have the same source, the Tao itself, and we are all equally divine beings. No matter how far we get in this life, if we treat others as we ourselves would like to be treated, take each day as it comes, and take the time to connect to our divine origin, we can live a successful and spiritually productive life.

By learning how to be our true selves and act in a spontaneous yet harmonious manner we can be of great assistance to the world around us. And we will find that people respond to us in a positive and joyful manner.

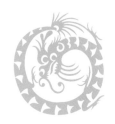

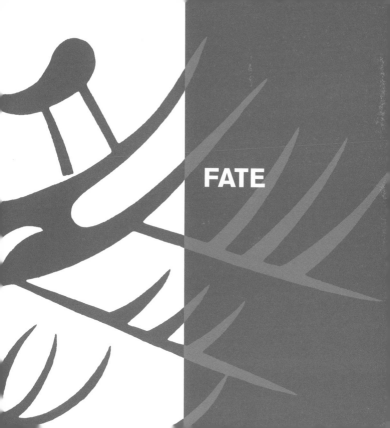

FATE

The Chinese believe that it is the life force that governs the universe, a sort of natural universal law that is created from itself and perpetuates, eternally. We humans are a part of that celestial force, what the Chinese call Tao. And, while there are certain factors that may appear to be random, they are also, in part, decided by our actions and aspirations in our lives.

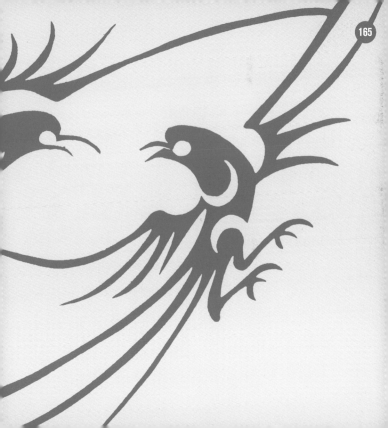

Some people believe that karma can extend from one lifetime to another. In other words, if you are guilty of moral or physical crimes in one life then you will suffer in the next. While this may be true to some extent, we also create new karma in every moment. Each decision made and action taken creates a new situation for us to deal with. It is our response then to that situation that creates new karma for us.

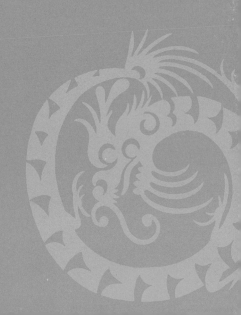

That which
happens without
man's causing it
to happen is
from fate.

WANG CHUNG

A Taoist considers things like "bad luck" or "bad dreams" merely as dramatic effects in his miraculous life.

HUA CHING NI

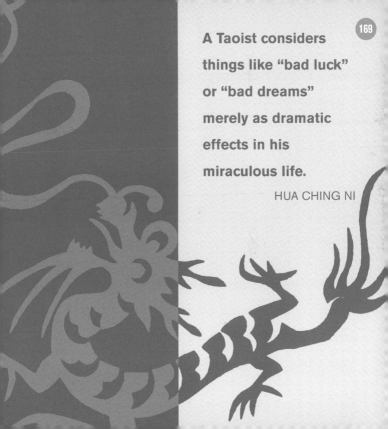

Heaven has no special feeling of kindness, but the greatest kindness comes from it by its being impartial to everything.

HUA CHING NI

Many people fall prey to seeing themselves as "victims" of fate, of bad luck, of other people's actions, of circumstance. They never see that their own actions and thoughts summon the bad fortune to them.

We have all certainly experienced forces in our lives that seem to be beyond our control. Things happen to us, seemingly at random, or for no reason at all that we can discern. Often we have actually set up those situations through our own actions, both in the past as well as in the present. We must remember that we are also living in a world filled with other people's karma or energetic forces.

172

The dynamics of any situation involve many different kinds of forces. While our experiences may be influenced by karma, astrology, or our own belief systems, often the only power we have is in our response to it in the moment it happens.

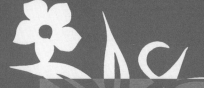

Fate is the force that interferes with our lives, wrecking things at the worst moments. Yet what we call fate is nothing more than the consequence of our own actions.

DENG MING DAO

Through our spiritual cultivation, it is possible to reach a state that is beyond time and space: what the ancients called "Attaining Tao." This is where past and future no longer have any influence upon us, when the only reality we experience is a continually unfolding present.

The sage places herself last,

Thus she is first.

She is not attached to her own life,

In this way her life is preserved.

Because she is selfless

She can attain fulfillment.

LAO TZU

People often believe that divination is simply predicting the future, or events that are bound to happen. Because of this misunderstanding, many people resign themselves to fate or destiny and do not see themselves as participants in the creation and dissolution of things.

EVA WONG

Everything is cyclical, and in every cycle there comes a point where things turn around. Great adversity was once overwhelming; now it starts to wane. Those who remain centered will go through bad times and eventually receive good fortune.

HUA CHING NI

Keep filling a vessel and it will overflow.

Oversharpen a blade and it will lose its edge.

If your house is full of gold and jade

It will be impossible to defend it.

To acquire wealth and fame in an arrogant fashion

Is to invite punishment.

Retire when your work is done.

This is the way of heaven.

LAO TZU

Doing things in a timely and appropriate fashion is an important step on the Path of Tao. Too much of anything is never a good thing, just as oversharpening a blade will cause it to lose its edge or overfilling a vessel will just create a big mess.

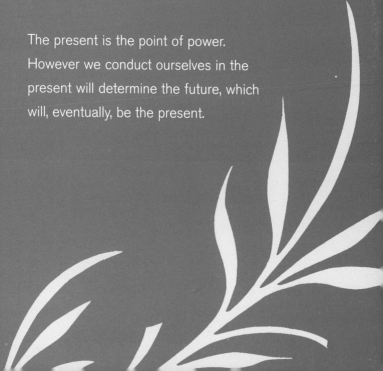

The present is the point of power. However we conduct ourselves in the present will determine the future, which will, eventually, be the present.

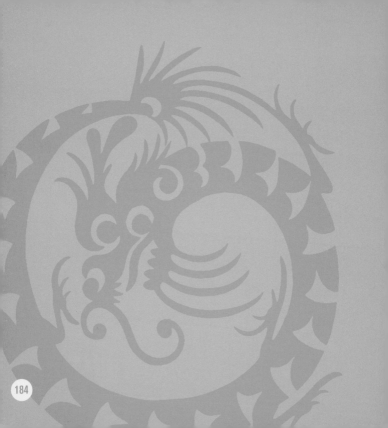

We all have our fate. Many of us have personal problems or even physical challenges that we were born with. It may seem very unfair for a newborn child to have to deal with health challenges when they are so innocent. Sometimes these things are the result of bad karma or negative energy residue from past lives, or perhaps they are the result of our own soul's attempt to learn certain life lessons.

All of us are born with certain strengths and weaknesses. We could call that our good or bad fortune. While there are things we can do to make it easier for our good fortune to flourish, we also need to learn how to function with whatever bad fortune we are given.

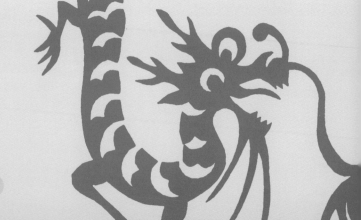

Regardless of the hand that fate has dealt us, there is always progress to be made. Often those who have to work the hardest to achieve success value it more and learn at a much deeper level than those who have an easy time and may not take life seriously.

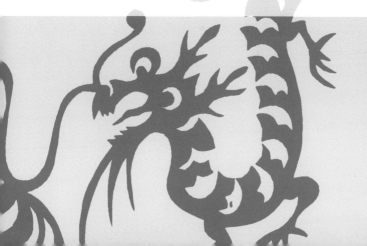

Some people need to work hard for everything they get. They are not as attractive or as healthy as others and have much more difficulty with life. Sometimes they are even abused when young and so grow up stunted or with deep emotional problems. It would seem that these people have a very unlucky fate.

Our empathy toward another person's misfortune is based on the assumption that if the same circumstances were to happen to us, we would feel bad and want to be pitied. Therefore, empathy may be based on self-pity rather than compassion toward others.

EVA WONG

We all live in our own sense of reality. What may be a positive experience to one person may be a negative experience for another. We can never judge another person by our own standards or understanding of a situation or communication. It may be entirely different.

Once a man by the name of Chi Liang suddenly fell ill. He went from bad to worse and seemed on the verge of death. So his sons sent for three doctors, fearing the worst. The first doctor looked at the patient and told him, "Your yin and yang are out of balance and your internal organs are out of order. Your illness is due to bad eating habits, too much sex, and too much worrying. With the proper care and rest you can be cured."

Chi Liang said, "He is only an average doctor. Send him away immediately!"

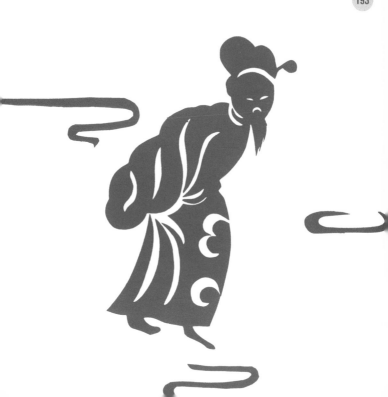

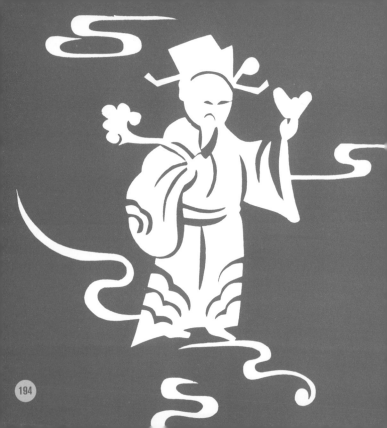

The second doctor felt the patient's pulses and looked at his tongue. "Your illness," he said, "is of a constitutional nature, due to insufficient nutrition from your mother's womb. While she may have nursed you well after you were born, the damage had already been done. I am afraid this illness has been building for a long time and is irreversible."

"This one is a good doctor," said Chi Liang. "Please invite him to stay for dinner."

The third doctor came in and took one look at his patient and said, "Your illness has not been caused by heaven, man, or from spirits. Each of us is endowed at birth with the life force. This is not something that can be controlled. There is no medicine that can help you now."

"This man is a divine doctor," said Chi Liang. "Reward him handsomely!"

Soon after this, Chi Liang's illness was cured by itself.

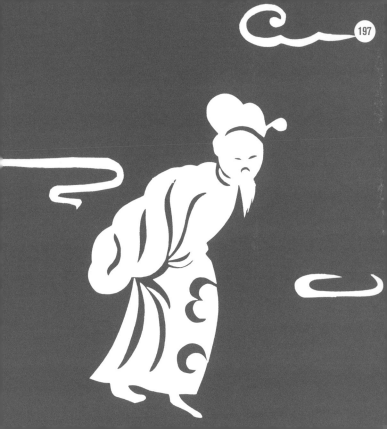

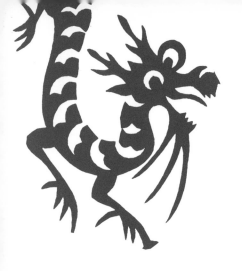

It is said that if you value your life too much you will lose it. If you are overattached to your health you will not be healthy. Then again, if you abuse yourself and do not take care of yourself you will also get sick and die. Our life, our death, health, and sickness, all of these come of themselves. We must learn to let nature take its own course. We can't make things happen and we should not try to prevent things from happening.

LIEH TZU

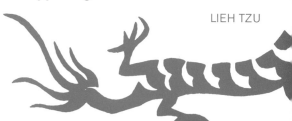

Accept disgrace willingly.

Accept misfortune as the human condition.

What do you mean by "Accept disgrace willingly?"

Accept being unimportant.

Do not be concerned with loss or gain.

This is called "accepting disgrace willingly."

LAO TZU

The ancient sages worried about favor as much as disgrace, because they knew that favor is followed by disgrace. Other people think favor means to go up, and disgrace means to go down. But favor cannot be separated from disgrace. Disgrace comes from favor.

SU CHE

Often there is no way to separate our joy from our suffering. They are often linked in some way. If we want to be open to joy, we must remain open to suffering.

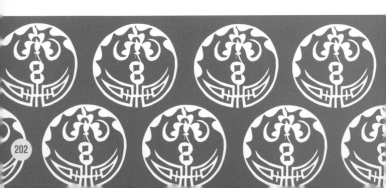

The Buddhists say all life is suffering. And while life certainly does contain its fair share of suffering, it is often balanced out by the joy, the excitement, and the simple pleasures that come our way. But to try and avoid all suffering will only create more suffering.

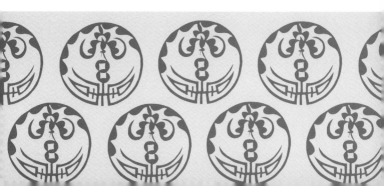

A person who has no spiritual knowledge themselves will not even see a sage for what he or she is. They will seem quite ordinary or even simple-minded.

Misfortune has built all the great sages. It was through great difficulties that they were enlightened. Do not depend on good fortune. Depend on your own virtuous personality and normal life to make you the final winner.

HUA CHING NI

We are all beautiful golden sunflowers, rising up out of the dark earth, blooming in the sun, shining on everyone and everything in all our golden sunflower glory, then fading back into the dark earth at the end of our season. This is our destiny; this is our fate. And it is just and natural and even beautiful that it be so. And in our death, we seed the earth so that more golden sunflowers may rise and in their beauty we will live again.

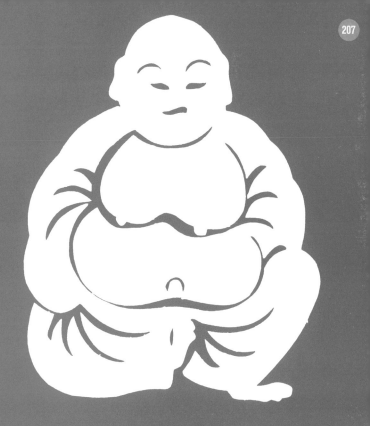

If we remember and are conscious that each day is a miracle unfolding, no matter how bad we feel, it is easier to keep things in perspective.

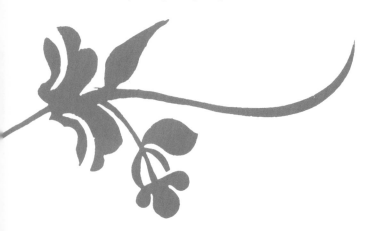

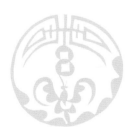

RIGHT TIMING:

THE *I CHING*

A large part of any successful venture is in the timing. Right timing, like right placement, has always been of great concern to Taoists. One of the tools they have utilized is the *I Ching* (*yi jing*) or *Book of Changes*. The *I Ching* is believed to be the oldest book on the planet.

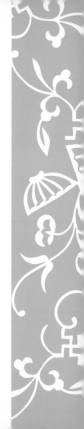

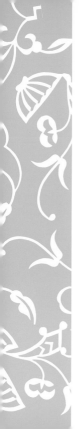

It is believed to have been devised by the ancient Taoist Immortal Fu Shi five thousand years ago. Three thousand years ago it was revised by King Wen and his son the Duke of Chou, founders of the Chou Dynasty. It was then edited and annotated by Confucius six hundred years later.

In ancient China, divination was conducted by heating the shells of tortoises which caused them to crack. The cracks were then read and interpreted. It was from these that Fu Shi developed his method of using broken and unbroken lines.

In 215 B.C.E., the tyrant emperor Chin Shih Huang Ti ordered a mass burning of books (and scholars!) but spared the *I Ching*.

In the *I Ching*, the trigrams (three lines) themselves are all based on natural elements such as water, mountain, wind, thunder, and earth. They also represent various human interactions, both with nature and society. The readings are created by combining two trigrams into a hexagram (six lines) and are often in the form of an allegory and need to be studied closely to reveal their wisdom. The more you reflect on the reading, the more you will learn.

The *I Ching* became so popular with scholars and sages in China that it has had a major influence on philosophy, statecraft, science, and medicine throughout China's history. Many rulers used the guidance of the *I Ching* when it came to making decisions about affairs of the state. Yet it can also be used for personal cultivation, reflection, or guidance by anyone. Whether you need to make a personal decision, a business decision, or just want some feedback from the Tao, the *I Ching* is the perfect tool for the job!

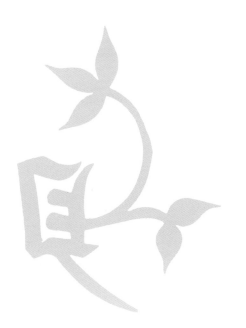

The *I Ching* uses the system of yin and yang. The yin/yang theory is the original binary system. By combining three and then six yin or yang lines, the *I Ching* is able to represent many different sets of reality, each one unique to a specific time and situation. Basically, the *I Ching* shows you all the forces that are working on a particular time, the present. The present is the point of power. It is in how we respond to those forces that are affecting this present moment that creates the future.

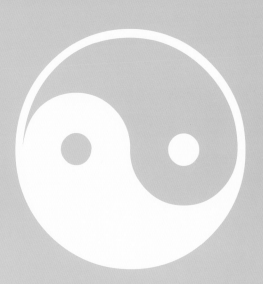

The main principle is that nothing remains static. Everything in nature is subject to perpetual change. However, this change occurs in regular cycles and is governed by certain immutable laws which, however, are flexible enough to permit wide scope for man to act for better or for worse. Therefore, if we penetrate the laws governing the movements of the universe, we can learn how things are going to happen; and; knowing that, we can learn how to adapt ourselves to each forthcoming situation.

JOHN BLOFELD

The Emperor's Dilemma:
An *I Ching* fable, part I

His August Presence, the Emperor, Son of Heaven, sat stiffly upon the Dragon Throne while his soothsayers and diviners knelt before him, trembling. The barbarian hordes were once again pressing on the north, teasing and nipping about the heels of his army, spread thinly along the Long Wall. To the south rebellious lords were muttering among themselves and were said to be massing armies to march upon the capital.

The question was, should he pull yet more troops from the south to send to the north or should he be doing the opposite, in case there was something to the rumors of rebellion? What to do?

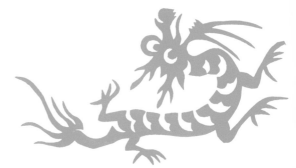

He looked down upon his trembling soothsayers, diviners, and counselors. Did they have the answer? His thoughts went back to the ragged Taoist that had recently come to the capital from his home in the wild and dangerous mountains. He had presented himself to the court, saying he would like to offer his services to the Emperor and was turned away immediately. Now the Emperor was having second thoughts about this man.

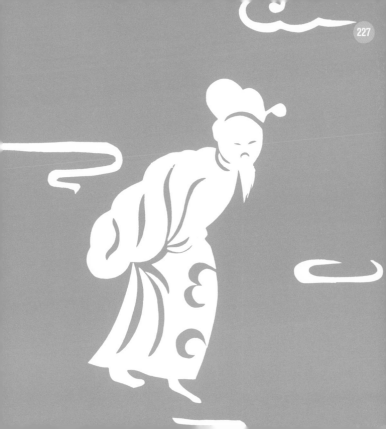

He called for his chief steward and gave him orders to send out guards and find the mountain man and bring him to the Forbidden City. It took three whole days but at last the ragged Taoist was found and brought to the Son of Heaven. He knelt before the throne with his head up and back straight while the Emperor looked at him thoughtfully.

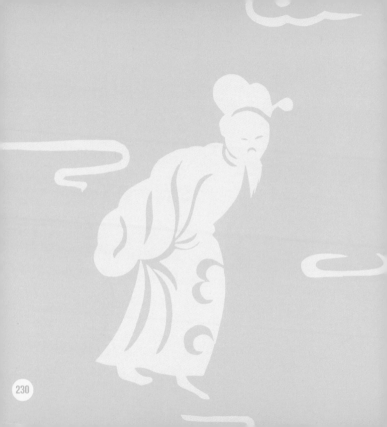

He was certainly a strange one, with his ragged clothing and long hair, knotted carelessly on top his head, and a long beard full of briars and twigs. Something about his bearing was almost royal despite skin like brown parchment and eyes like wildfires.

The Emperor's Dilemma:
An *I Ching* fable, part II

After what seemed like the proper time had passed, the Emperor spoke. "I have much on my mind at this time. I am in need of counsel. I have heard that you have offered your wisdom to serve your Emperor."

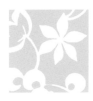

"That is true," was all the man said. The Emperor was tempted to have him thrown out on his ear, if not flogged with bamboo canes, for his insolent manner but stopped himself. "What is it that you use for your divination?" he asked.

"A book, your majesty," was the answer.

"It must be a very special book," said the Emperor.

"Yes, sire it is a very special book."

"Well, let's have a look at this very special book then."

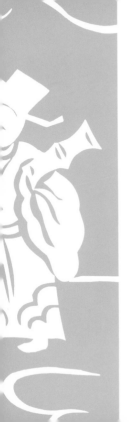

The mountain sage reached into his ragged robes and pulled forth a book, covered in red silk. "This, sire," he said, laying the book on the floor before him, "is called *The Book of Changes*."

"I have heard of this book," said the Emperor, peering down at it, "but have never seen it. How does it work?"

Here the Taoist opened the book and, pointing to one of the pages, said, "Here you see two lines, one broken in the middle, one unbroken. They represent the yin force and the yang force. The yin line represents the downward, inward force while the yang line represents the upper, outward force. These two lines represent the constant interaction and interdependence of all life."

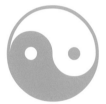

The Emperor's Dilemma:
An *I Ching* fable, part III

Here the Taoist produced three coins of the lowest denomination. "There is no need for expensive or rare coins," he said. He held them out to the Emperor, who, after craning his neck to see them, suddenly got down from his throne and sat on the floor opposite the sage.

"Notice that one side of the coins are inscribed and the other is not. We will call the inscribed side the yin side and the uninscribed side the yang. We take the coins like this."

He held them in his palm and closed his hand over them, shook them, and suddenly dropped them to the floor.

"Everything in the universe contains and is contained within this system of yin and yang. Every situation calls for a strong forward movement or its opposite. It is important to know when to move forward and when to retreat and when to just sit still and let the interplaying forces sort themselves out before moving at all."

"Yes," cried the Emperor excitedly, "this is what I need to know. How does it work?" The coins fell at the Emperor's feet with two inscribed sides up and one inscribed side down. "This gives us a yin line," said the Taoist. "We will do this six times and in that way be given a hexagram and a reading connected to that hexagram. There are sixty-four possible combinations of six yin and yang lines. Each combination gives us a different picture and a different reading."

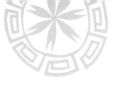

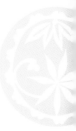

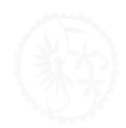

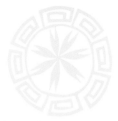

"Sire," said the Taoist, "now you must meditate on the problem set before you. You must cleanse yourself of all thinking and judgment, open yourself to the voice of the oracle, and promise the guiding spirits that you will listen without reservation. Only then will you be able to make full use of it."

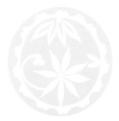

The system of hexagrams which we call
the *Book of Changes* or *I Ching* was one
of the first great successes
in ancient man's attempts to find the
laws which regulate all phenomena.

HUA CHING NI

When one faces a new situation, his mind is often on the past. This kind of thinking creates obstacles to an accurate, intuitive response which is more important than a conceptual understanding of the situation.

HUA CHING NI

You might think of the *I Ching* as a tool for connecting to your higher power. Information is available to us all the time through what we might call our spiritual self or higher power. Yet most of the time we have so much static going on in our heads that we cannot access this information. By quieting our hearts and minds, we are better able to quiet down the static and noise that we usually carry with us and are better able to hear that "still small voice within."

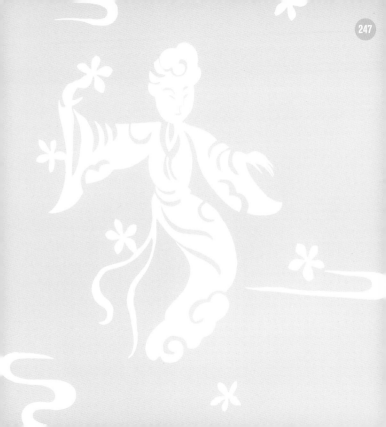

The Emperor's Dilemma:
An *I Ching* fable, part IV

The Taoist then handed the coins to the Emperor,
and the Son of Heaven took them in trembling
hands. There was so much at stake: the safety and
order of an entire nation and the Middle Kingdom
itself. How could this book look into his heart and
into the conflicting thoughts and make sense out
of them?

"How can this work?" he asked. "How do my
hands know which coins to throw?"

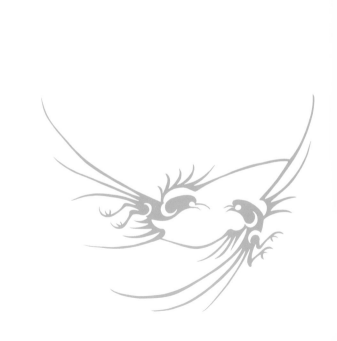

"That is simple, my lord," answered the Taoist. "Your hands are merely the means to unlock the knowledge that you yourself already have, buried deep within yourself. The spirit of the oracle will unlock those doors and let the treasure out. Then you will have the knowledge that you seek.

"The important thing to remember, my lord, is that it is one thing to know what the future holds, but another thing entirely to respond appropriately to that knowledge. You must use all the wisdom and experience of your years to respond positively and decisively, once the oracle has revealed itself to you.

"At any moment, there are many forces or patterns converging," the Taoist went on. "How we respond and work with these is what creates the future and our role in it. By becoming sensitive to those patterns we can foretell the future and influence creating it. This is the true wisdom of the oracle."

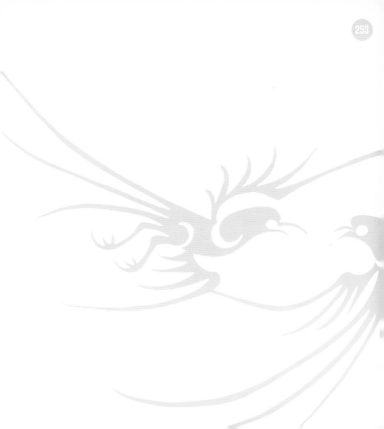

The Emperor's Dilemma:
An *I Ching* fable, part V

Here the Emperor took several more deep, slow breaths, closed his hand upon the coins, and, after shaking them a moment, threw them down on the carpet in front of him. They showed one inscribed and two uninscribed sides up.

"That gives us a yang or unbroken line," said the Taoist. He then produced a roll of cheap paper, brush, and ink. After slowly grinding a small amount of ink, he dipped the brush into the ink and wrote an unbroken line at the bottom of the paper.

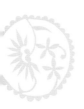

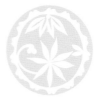

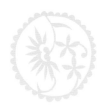

Again the Emperor shook and threw the coins. Again, they came up with one inscribed and two uninscribed sides up.

"Another yang line," said the Taoist and, dipping his brush once again, he drew another unbroken line, this time above the one he had already written.

Three more times the Emperor threw the coins and each time they came up the same, until the sage had drawn five unbroken lines on the paper, one on top of the other. Then, on the sixth throw, the coins lay with all three inscribed sides up.

"Ah," said the Taoist, "that is an old yin line, or a moving line, that will lead us to a whole other hexagram, which will give some foreshadowing on the future, if you respond to the first hexagram in the most felicitous way, of course."

The Taoist then picked up the oracle itself and, after consulting a diagram of trigrams, wrote down the number of the hexagram the Emperor had received, number forty three, *Kuai* or *Breaks Through*, sometimes called *Determination*.

"Here you have chosen *Tui*, the *Joyous* or *The Lake* over *Ch'ien*, the *Creative* or *Heaven*. It is a most auspicious reading."

I Ching practice enables one to discern good fortune from bad fortune in any situation and to respond appropriately with a good positive attitude. You, yourself, become the main factor for changing your future and destiny.

HUA CHING NI

The Emperor's Dilemma:
An *I Ching* fable, part VI

The Emperor then eagerly listened as the Taoist read to him the judgment. "Determination dissolves evil forces. One should obtain the cooperation of all righteous forces. Isolated and hasty actions are inappropriate. The advancement of cooperative, virtuous energy is wise."

The Taoist looked up at the Son of Heaven and said, "This hexagram is often compared to a breakthrough after a long accumulation of tension, like a swollen river breaking through its dikes or a sudden cloudburst. It also signifies a time when inferior people will gradually begin to disappear. Their insolence is on the wane, as a result of resolute action."

"It is important to remember that you cannot fight evil directly," continued the Taoist. "It will be ineffective and will cause you harm. You must find a way to approach the problem indirectly, but with firmness and resolution based on a union of strength and friendliness. It is a difficult path but it will most benefit the kingdom."

"Also," said the Taoist, looking at the Son of Heaven directly in his eyes, something which no commoner had ever done before, "you must look deeply into your own heart and find and uproot the evil and disease that dwells there so that you will be pure enough to rule wisely and justly."

The Emperor's Dilemma:
An *I Ching* fable, part I

The Emperor bowed his head, something that he had never done to any man. "I understand," was all he said.

"Now, as to the old yin or changing line. It tells us that danger is present. As I said before, evil cannot be challenged directly. It will only feed on force and finally overwhelm you. Instead you must use *wu wei* or nonaction.

Do not presume to attack evil head on. Instead, cultivate yourself and you will become strong enough and wise enough to know when evil is afoot and be able to eradicate it before it grows too strong."

"I understand," said the Emperor, humbly. "And what of the second reading?"

The Taoist smiled widely and showed the Emperor the next reading. It was the Dragon, the first hexagram in the oracle, Heaven over Heaven. "Indeed, this is most auspicious" he said.

"This reading", continued the Taoist, "shows us that if your lordship follows the advice of the previous reading then all will be well. You will not only save the kingdom but be at one with the Tao and become a sage ruler and be remembered for all time."

Long after the Taoist had left, the Emperor sat on the carpet in the dimming light, pondering what had been revealed to him. He felt a great opening in his soul and a smaller beginning of wisdom stirring within him.

For many years after that he was able to find guidance and wisdom in the oracle, which the Taoist had so kindly left him. He ruled justly and prudently and never neglected his own cultivation, even as he cultivated his kingdom. He did indeed become a sage ruler as was foretold and he passed into history as one of the great emperors of all time.

It is said that after one uses the *I Ching* for
many years, and applied oneself to meditation
and stilling the chatter of the mind, one doesn't
even need the *I Ching* to get information; it will
be readily available to you at any time.

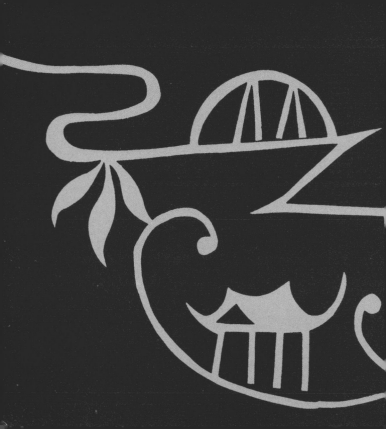

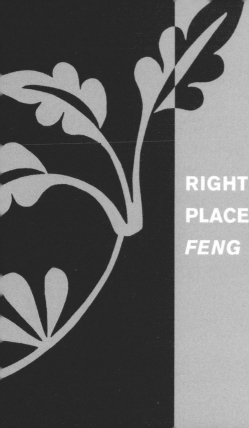

RIGHT
PLACEMENT:
FENG SHUI

Feng shui, pronounced "fung shway," is the Taoist art of wind and water, or right placement. It has its origins thousands of years ago. It can be traced back to the ancient Chinese shamans. Then, Taoist diviners, magicians, and scholars all developed it into a systematic science. Today, *feng shui* is considered to be one of the great practical arts of Taoism.

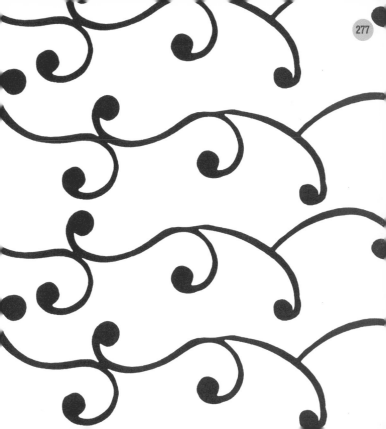

The first practitioners of what we today call *feng shui* were probably the *fang shih* (Masters of Prescriptions). The *fang shih*, sometimes referred to as Taoist magicians, were men and women who were experts in such things as astrology, astronomy, spirit healing, divination, and geomancy. They used herbal formulations, talismans, *chi gong* exercises, meditation, and invocations. During the Han dynasty, the imperial court kept *fang shih* on hand for their knowledge of astrology, divination, healing, and the arts of longevity.

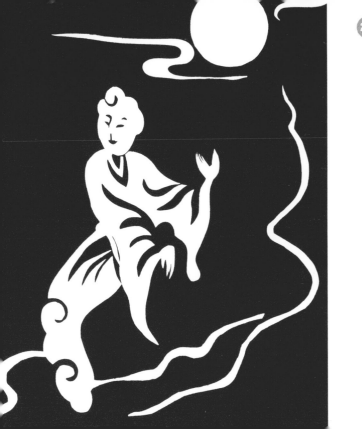

Modern *feng shui* masters still use the concepts developed by the ancient Taoists to improve energy flow, "lighten up" the energetic atmosphere, create good fortune, allow the free flow of wealth and good health in a living or working environment, and generally improve the energetic health of a building or room.

For centuries, the Chinese people have relied on *feng shui* to design cities, build homes, and bury their dead.

EVA WONG

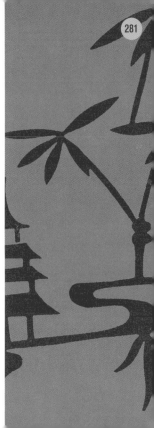

By recognizing *chi* in a landscape, the ancient ones determined which locations would be safe from danger, provide lush vegetation, or harmoniously align with the geomagnetism of the earth.

SUSAN LEVITT

One of the basic principles of *feng shui* is that we, as humans, are not the center of the universe.

Lao Tzu speaks of the interrelationship of all things. It is in studying the relationships of the elements, directions, colors, landforms, waterways, and the balance of yin and yang aspects of any building, room, or endeavor that *feng shui* is able to be of assistance.

An auspicious site is one where the vital energy called Ch'i flowed in a manner that was harmonious and supportive of human life.

How many times have you walked into a building, or even a room, and felt a sense of dread or foreboding or perhaps just a general sense of being uncomfortable there? It may have not been from anything that you could accurately lay a finger on, just a sense of unease. This feeling could orginate from the negative energy of a violent crime committed in the area or an awkward room layout.

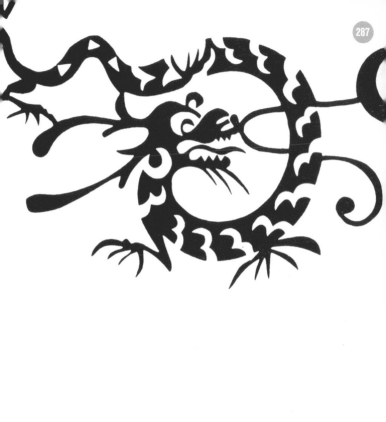

An ideal building location would be on even ground, and protected on back and sides by hills, mountains, or a forest. In front would be water—a river, a stream, a lake, or even a pond, which of course could be artificially built.

According to *feng shui*, our life and destiny are closely interwoven with the workings of the universe and nature.

SARAH ROSSBACH

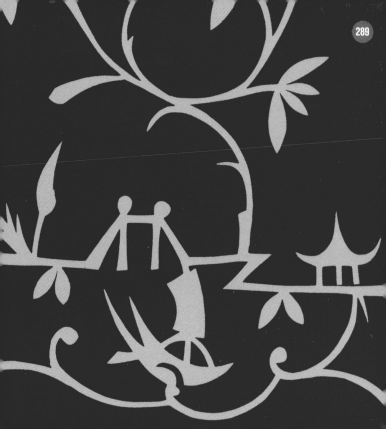

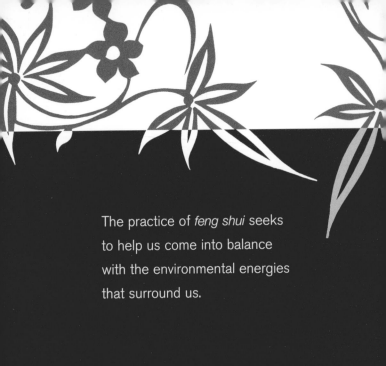

The practice of *feng shui* seeks
to help us come into balance
with the environmental energies
that surround us.

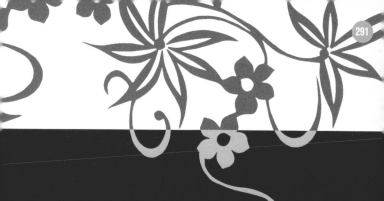

Harmony and balance are both crucial factors in *feng shui*—they pervade the process linking man and the universe. And that process is called Tao.

SARAH ROSSBACH

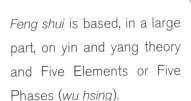

Feng shui is based, in a large part, on yin and yang theory and Five Elements or Five Phases (*wu hsing*).

The qualities held by yin are darkness, water, cold, rest, inward and downward direction, stillness, receptivity, and what we think of as femaleness.

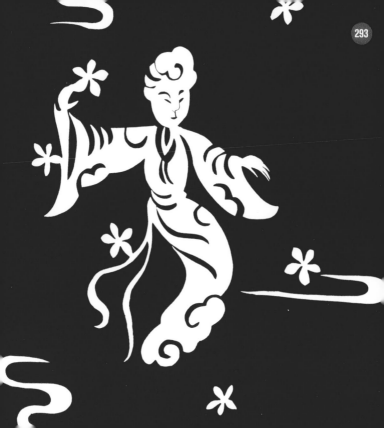

The qualities of yang are brightness, heat, activity, upward and outward direction, aggressiveness, expansion, and what we think of as maleness.

The wood element corresponds to the color green—
the green of new growth, of grasses and plants—and
to the liver. Its direction is east and the season spring.

The fire element corresponds to the color red, to the heart, the direction of south, and the season of summer, when the fiery sun is at its highest aspect.

The earth element corresponds to the color yellow, the direction of the center and the season of Indian summer or the time between seasons. It is where we feel our connection to the earth.

The metal or gold element corresponds to the color white, the lungs, the direction of west, and the season of autumn.

The water element corresponds to
the color blue-black, the kidneys,
the direction north, and the season
of winter.

The wood element symbolizes the energy of growth, or the generating phase.

The fire element symbolizes expansion, or the fully grown phase.

The earth element symbolizes the
energy of rooting and centering,
or the harmonizing phase.

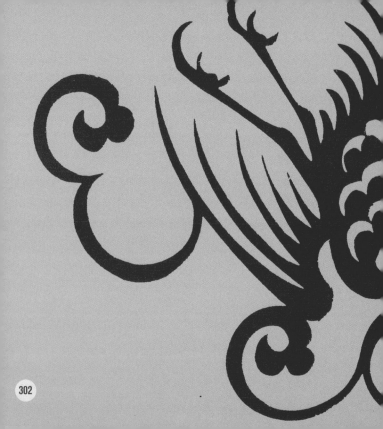

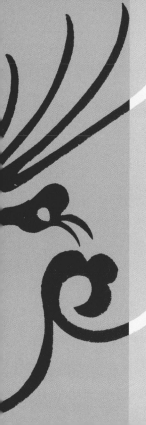

The metal or gold element symbolizes the energy of contraction and gathering, or the introverting phase.

The water element symbolizes the energy returning to the source, or the root phase.

The five elements—water, gold, earth, wood, and fire—work together in different cycles. These are the nourishing cycle, the controlling cycle, and the reducing cycle.

In the nourishing cycle, wood feeds fire, fire creates earth, earth contains metal, metal holds water, and water feeds wood. This can be seen using the natural metaphors of wood burning in a fire, fire creating ash, ash being used in smelting to produce metal, metal being formed into a container for water, and then water being used to nourish plants.

The controlling cycle works like this: Fire controls metal, metal controls wood, wood controls earth, earth controls water, and water controls fire. Another way to look at it is fire melting metal, metal cutting wood, wood penetrating earth, earth damming water, and water extinguishing fire.

306

In the reducing cycle, fire burns wood, wood (like the roots of a tree) sucks up water, water rusts metal, metal is taken from the earth, and earth suffocates fire.

We would use the nourishing cycle to balance the elements in a specific building or room.

Generally, it is the shapes, colors and materials of furnishings and decorative objects that affect the flow of *chi* energy.

SIMON BROWN

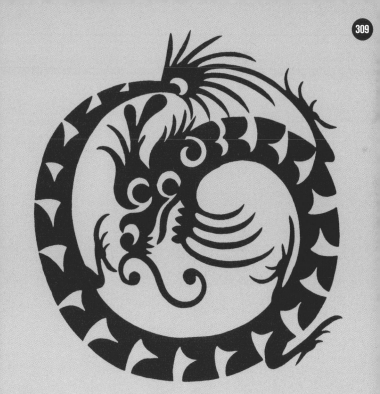

If we want to add an element of water to the room, we can use fountains or aquariums.

If the room is too yang, or bright, then we can add some plants, utilizing the wood element, to control or balance the fire that is predominant.

If the room is overloaded with the wood element—wood floor, heavy beams, etc.—we can use the metal element to balance it by using a white or light rug on the floor, painting the walls white, or using light fabric on the furniture.

Feng shui considers the specific use of the space and who is going to be using it. Sometimes you may want to have a more dark and watery atmosphere, say in a place where you will be resting or meditating. Another space may be used for exercise or other high energy use so it would be fine for it to be very bright. We must try to avoid bland generalities in *feng shui* and keep in mind that we want different kinds of energies in different kinds of spaces.

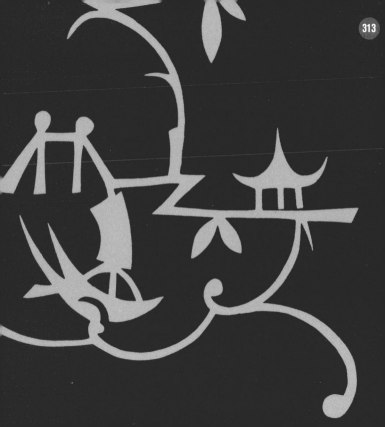

The character or elemental makeup of the person using the space is important in *feng shui*. A high-energy, slightly manic type of person may need to work or live in a space that will mute his or her fiery energy. They will need to add some earth elements to their space. Another person may be a low-energy, slow-moving type and will need to utilize some fire or bright energy in their space to help them achieve balance.

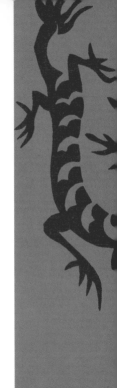

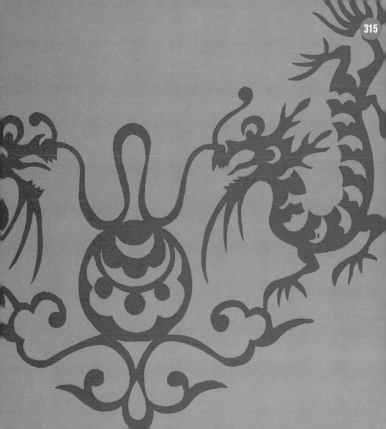

Light sources are very important when designing a space. Strong or soft light, the direction it is coming from, whether it is natural or electric lighting —all have different effects on the space and even the *chi* of the room.

Try to keep computers out of the sleeping or resting area, especially if you tend to leave them on. When you do use a computer, sit far enough away from the monitor to reduce health risks or use a screen.

Before you do anything to a space, spend some time there and imagine yourself either working or relaxing there to see what kinds of feelings that brings up. It is important to remember that different people respond to different elements in different ways, depending on their own elemental makeup. Then, try different things until you feel that you have achieved an elemental harmony that works for you.

Taoist observation of Nature concluded that curved, flowing lines slow *chi* and bring abundance. Harmonious *chi* moves in a curved, graceful line, as if following the natural course of a river. Sharp, straight lines bring *sha chi*, or bad *chi*.

SUSAN LEVITATE

It is believed by *feng shui* masters that *chi* or abundant good fortune will flow too quickly through an area that is too open, such as a room with a window opposite a door, or another door. It is believed that the energy will flow in through the door and right out again through the window or opposite door.

A negative situation would be a room with only one door and no windows. The energy or *chi* would flow in through the door and then circle endlessly through the room, bringing confusion and disorientation.

To practice *Feng Shui* today, we need to blend traditional *Feng Shui* wisdom with our own keen intuitive, investigative, diagnostic, and communicative skills.

TERAH KATHRYN COLLINS

The balance of yin and yang in the home or office is important. A dark, musty room full of heavy furniture will not be inviting for other people or good energy.

On the other hand, a too-bright, empty room with sharp corners everywhere will also not be conducive to comfort and ease.

The ancient shaman-kings'
mastery of the elements can also
be attributed to their knowledge of
landforms and weather.

EVA WONG

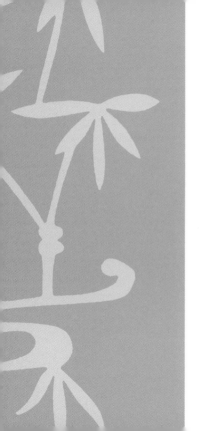

There are different styles of *feng shui* today. You can try experimenting with several styles to find the one that feels the best for you and your situation. Having a positive attitude and a harmonious spirit will be of great assistance to your life, regardless of your environment.

The true learning of *feng shui* begins when we acknowledge our place in the universe, not necessarily a dominant place, but one that has its role in the scheme of things.

EVA WONG

The study of *feng shui* begins with understanding the presence of the Tao in nature and in humanity.

EVA WONG

There are many things you can use to counter any negative flow of *chi* in a room or building. One of these is a mirror. *Feng shui* masters believe mirrors to be capable of reflecting or deflecting *chi*. Another "cure" is the use of windchimes or lamps. Plants, either living or artificial, can also be used. For more detailed explanation on how to use these objects consult a book on *Feng shui* or, better yet, a *Feng shui* master.

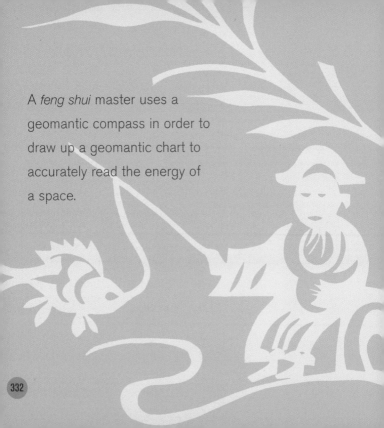

A *feng shui* master uses a geomantic compass in order to draw up a geomantic chart to accurately read the energy of a space.

Authentic *Feng Shui* does not have fixed rules of when to do things or where to put objects. Instead, it relies on a deep understanding of the patterns of energy in the universe and their interactions with the individual.

LAM KAM CHUEN

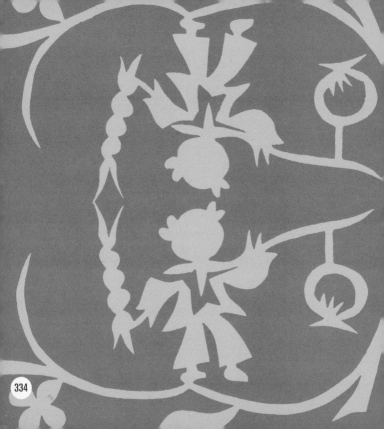

A basic ingredient of *feng shui* is the *ba gua* or eight-sided map. Each *gua*, or section, corresponds to an area of your life. Beginning at the north (on the bottom of the Chinese map) and moving round the room from the left, the life-areas are career, knowledge, family, wealth, fame, relationships, children, and helpful people. How you set up each section of the room will have an effect on that area of your life. Thus, bad *chi* or inharmonious effects in that section of space will have a negative effect on that area of your life.

The art of *feng shui* is to balance all five elements in a harmonious way.

SUSAN LEVITT

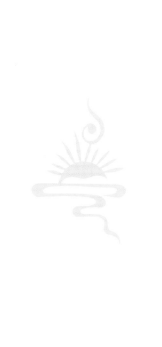

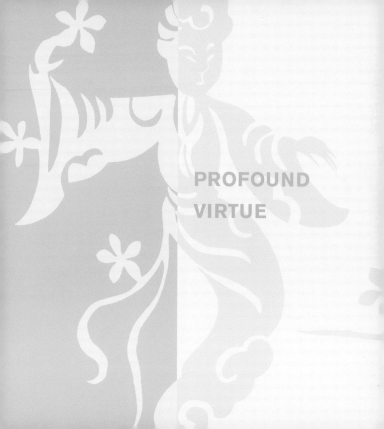

PROFOUND
VIRTUE

The word for virtue in Chinese is *te*, pronounced "*de*." Yet the term *te* means much more than what we might think of as virtue in the West. It can also be thought of as power or personal power. It is a power that we are all born with but which few of us choose to develop. A great part of self-cultivation is to develop and enhance our *te*.

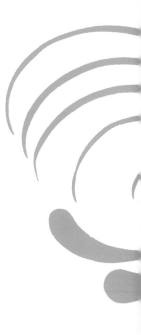

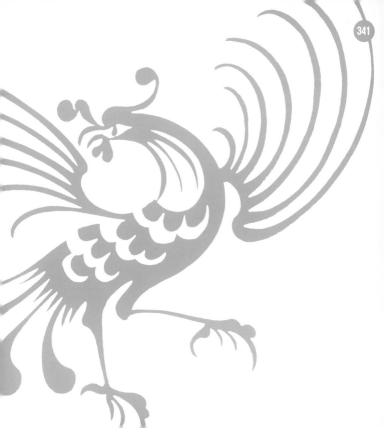

In ancient times, it was thought that emperors and other nobility had more *te* than the common people, though they had to observe special rites and rituals to preserve and enhance it.

Mountains and other high places were also thought to have great amounts of natural *te* and so people climbed them at special times, such as on the ninth day of the ninth month, to absorb the most beneficial *te*.

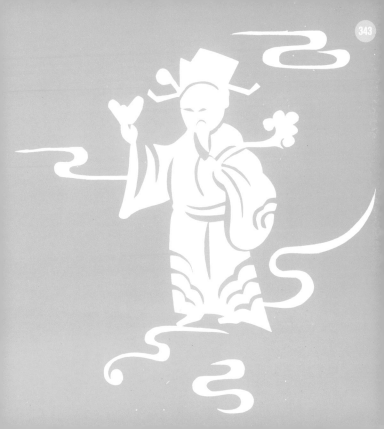

Rocks, plants, animals, and the whole natural world was thought to contain *te*. The *orenda* or *wakan* of the Native Americans, the *pneuma* of the Greeks, and the "holy spark" of the Hasidic Jews are all examples of this amorphous yet powerful substance or quality.

Virtue implies a oneness with the Tao, an ability to act in harmony with the universe. Profound Virtue is that quality seen in sages; men and women who have cultivated themselves so that they can act in perfect harmony in any situation, invoking the natural compassion of the universe.

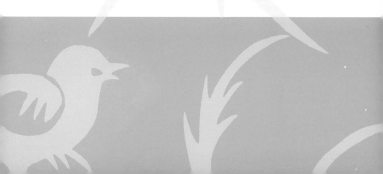

To be moral is to be virtuous, to be virtuous is to be natural, to be natural is to be one with the unending cycles of the Tao. Profound Virtue is unconscious virtue. In other words, it is who you are, not what you do.

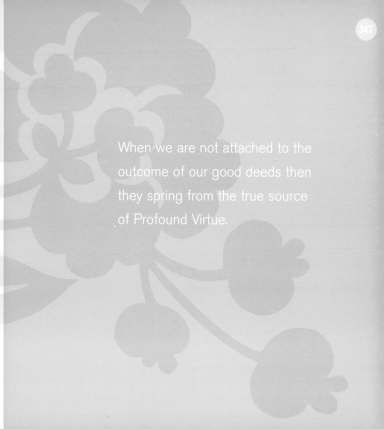

When we are not attached to the
outcome of our good deeds then
they spring from the true source
of Profound Virtue.

The Chinese word for *te* contains the symbol for movement on the left. On the right are the symbols for an eye and the heart.

Te is, in a sense, Tao made manifest, the revelation of the true nature of the Tao.

J.C. COOPER

Te is sometimes translated as personal power. It is a type of spiritual and energetic power that comes from people who are at peace with themselves.

Te can be cultivated, fostered, and used to attract other people, spiritual powers, even economic prosperity.

The Tao gives birth to all things

But Virtue nourishes them,

Furthers them, lets them grow,

Raises them and ripens them,

Fosters them and protects them.

To give birth is not to possess.

To act without directing,

This is called Profound Virtue.

LAO TZU

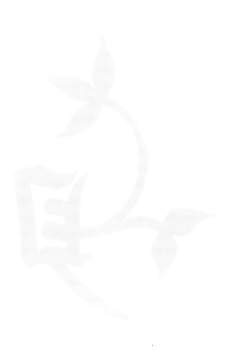

By taking care of our own personal virtue, we are actually affecting the virtue of others, perhaps making it easier for them to pursue their own sense of personal virtue.

Among the ten thousand things

All honor the Tao and esteem Virtue.

This is not because it is commanded,

But because it is our nature.

LAO TZU

Cultivate Virtue in yourself,

And Virtue will be true.

Cultivate it in your family

And the family's Virtue will be plentiful.

Cultivate it in the village,

And the Virtue of the village will be long lasting.

Cultivate it in the nation,

And the Virtue of the nation will be abundant.

Cultivate it in all things under heaven,

And Virtue will be universal.

LAO TZU

When we are authentic and unconscious of our virtue, seeking no reward and fearing no punishment, then we can be said to have attained Profound Virtue.

The one who has Profound Virtue is
like an infant.
Poisonous insects will not sting her;
Fierce beasts will not seize her;
Birds of prey will not attack her.

LAO TZU

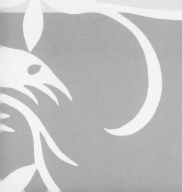

To be virtuous is to be pure, even innocent. This can feel like a liability in our troubled world. But ultimately, it will contribute to our liberation.

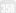

Virtue establishes a close connection between ourselves and the external world. Each of us should seek harmony with everyone and everything, at any time, anywhere.

YAN XIN

Lung Shu went to see the physician Wen Chih and said, "I have heard that your abilities are great and subtle. I have an illness I was hoping you could cure."

"Your wish is my command," said Wen Chih. "Please tell me of your symptoms."

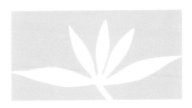

"Well," began Lung Shu, "I do not feel it is an honor if the whole district praises me, nor do I think it a disgrace if the whole state reviles me. I do not feel joy when I win, nor do I feel anxiety if I lose. I feel the same way about life and death, riches and poverty, men and pigs, myself and others. I live in my own house as if I were lodging in an inn. I look at my own neighborhood as if it were a foreign and barbarous land."

Lung Shu continued. "Having all these systems, titles, and rewards do not interest me. Punishments and fines do not scare me Prosperity and decline, benefit and harm—none of these things can change me. Neither joy nor sorrow seem to influence me. Because of all of this it is impossible for me to serve my lord properly, have relations with my family and friends, manage my wife and children, or even control my servants. What sort of illness is this, and can you cure it?"

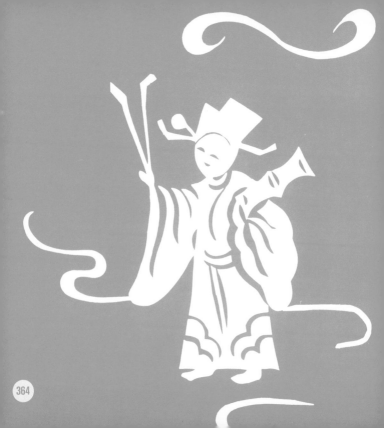

Wen Chih had Lung Shu stand in the window, with his back to the light. He then stepped back and looked at Lung Shu for a long time. Finally he sighed and said, "I see what your problem is. It is your heart. The center place is empty, you are almost a sage. While six of the holes of your heart run into one another, one is stopped up. This must be the reason you think that having the wisdom of a sage is an illness. I am afraid there is nothing I can do about it."

LIEH TZU

The truly virtuous among us may find it difficult to live in the world of dog-eat-dog. They may find it hard to conduct themselves in the world of high commerce and find fault with themselves for their seeming lack of ability.

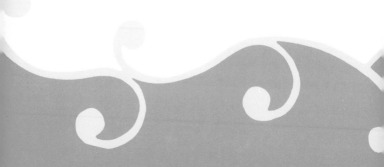

The truly virtuous may not be recognized by the
rest of the world, who may see them as weak
or foolish.

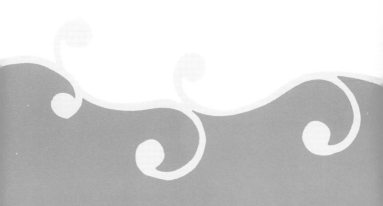

It is easy to be virtuous or kind and compassionate when we are feeling strong and healthy. But it is not so easy when we ourselves are feeling in need of kindness and compassion. Perhaps this is why the ancients used the term Profound Virtue.

To be successful, to be happy, to be healthy in mind and spirit, we need to cultivate virtue in our lives.
Merely considering oneself, relatives and friends is small virtue.
To be only concerned with the effects and interest at hand are also considered small virtues.

YAN XIN

This "virtue" has no moral overtones; it is an inward quality in man and all creatures, a potentiality and lent natural power arising from and dependent on the Tao, from which it is an emanation.

J.C. COOPER

The Tao gives birth to all things.

It is Virtue that nourishes them.

LAO TZU

What most people consider virtuous conduct may only be a sort of false modesty, a type of righteousness based on external principles, rather than those based on being in touch with your own natural, essential nature.

Our society has become highly unnatural and its citizens ever more cut off from their natural selves. It is no wonder that a common sense of virtue is being lost?

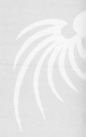

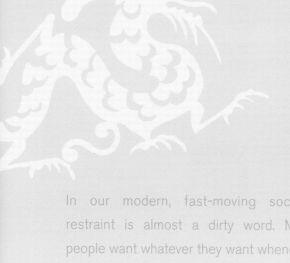

In our modern, fast-moving society, restraint is almost a dirty word. Most people want whatever they want whenever they want it, regardless of the destructive influence it may have on them, the planet, or society as a whole.

When governing people and serving Heaven

There is nothing like restraint.

Restraint is also called "being prepared early."

Being prepared early can be called

accumulation of Virtue.

When one continually accumulates Virtue

There is nothing that cannot be done.

LAO TZU

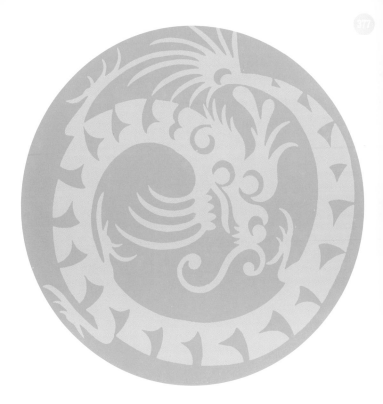

She who follows the Tao is one with the Tao;

She who is Virtuous is one with Virtue.

Those who lose the Tao are one with loss;

As for those who are at one with the Tao,

The Tao extends itself to them.

As for those who are at one with Virtue,

Virtue extends itself to them.

LAO TZU

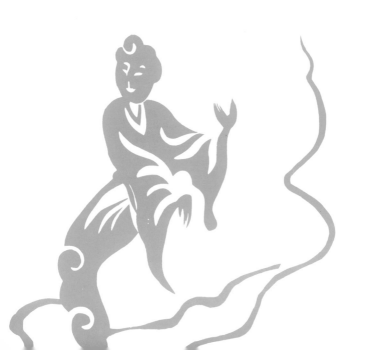

The greatest Virtue is to follow
the Tao and the Tao alone.

LAO TZU

Profound Virtue is deep;
It travels far;
It helps all things return to the Tao.

LAO TZU

By quieting the mind and heart and letting what is true, what is real, what is everlasting reside there, we can respond to any situation or person from our highest nature.

Yierh Tzu went to see Hsu Yu. Hsu Yu asked Yierh Tzu what he had learned from his teacher, master Yao.

"Master Yao has taught me that I must work at benevolence and righteousness and then I will be able to clearly discriminate between right and wrong."

"Then why have to come to me?" asked Hsu Yu. "Yao has already branded you with his sense of benevolence and righteousness, and has cut off your nose with his own ideas of right and wrong. How will you ever be able to wander on the path of aimless enjoyment, transcending ideas of right and wrong?"

"That may be," said Yierh Tzu, "but I would like to travel along its edges."

"I am sorry but that cannot be," said Hsu Yu. "A blind man cannot appreciate beauty in others. He who is sightless cannot distinguish the colors between various robes."

"Yes, well," said Yierh Tzu, "when Wu Chang lost her beauty, when Chu Liang lost his great strength, when the Yellow Emperor renounced his wisdom—these were all due to the process of reworking and remolding. How can you know but that the Creator of All Life may not take away my branding, give me back my nose? In this way I will become whole again and fit to be your student."

"It is true that you never can tell," answered Hsu Yu. "But my teacher, ah, my teacher. He gives to all who have need but does not consider it 'righteousness.' He gives favors that reach for generations but does not consider himself 'benevolent.' He is as old as antiquity but does not consider himself an elder. His goodness covers heaven and supports the earth, yet he does not consider himself "good." This is who you should follow."

CHUANG TZU

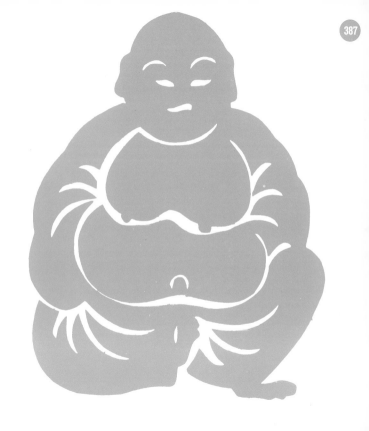

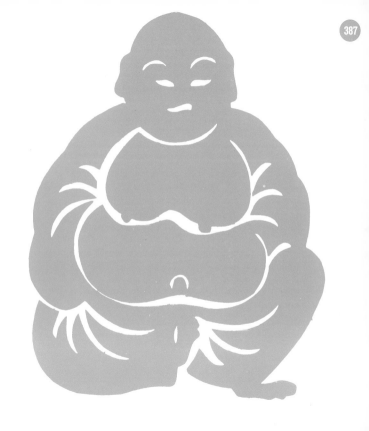

387

Remember that what other people call goodness and righteousness may have nothing to do with natural virtue. Real virtue must come from the inside, not from what society calls goodness.

Know honor
yet preserve humility.
Be as a valley for all
things under heaven.
By serving as a valley for
all things under heaven,
Allow the Unchanging
Virtue to be complete.

LAO TZU

To do right is to obey the laws of Nature, of Virtue, and to live in conformity and harmony with them. Failure to do so brings automatic and equally natural retribution, disharmony, disruption and consequent misery.

J.C. COOPER

When we try to go against
the laws of Nature, of virtue,
it is like spitting into the
wind. We will always get it
back in our face!

Lieh Tzu was studying with the Immortal Shang. After three years, he was no longer concerned with right and wrong, he no longer spoke of benefit and harm. It was only then that he got so much as a glance from Immortal Shang.

Then, after five years, he began once more to think of right and wrong; he began speaking of benefit and harm. It was then that Immortal Shang began to smile.

After seven years, he allowed whatever thought he had come into his mind without distinguishing between right and wrong. He said whatever came out of his mouth, no longer distinguishing between benefit and harm. It was then that Immortal Shang drew him to his side.

After nine years, he thought his own thoughts and spoke his own mind, without discriminating whether they were right and wrong, had benefit or harm; they were his own thoughts and words.

It was only then, after he had come to the end of everything inside him as well as outside him that his eyes became as his ears, his ears as his nose, his nose as his mouth.

It was all the same. His mind was calm and concentrated, his body relaxed, his bones and flesh fused completely. He did not notice where he stood or where he sat, what his mind was thinking about or what his words contained.

If we could all be like this, nothing will be hidden from us.

LIEH TZU

Because it is empty, the sage's mind can receive. Because it is still, it can respond.

HUI TSANG

Those who open themselves up to the Great Way, though their eyes see good and bad, their minds distinguish no difference. They don't treat the bad with goodness out of pity but because they don't perceive any difference.

WANG PANG

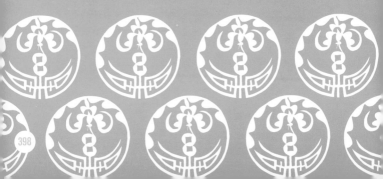

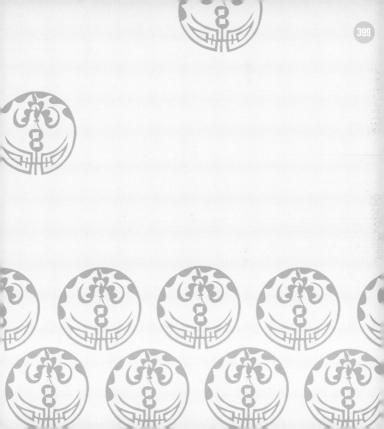

Profound Virtue is the perfect cultivation of the harmony of nature. Even if Virtue is not manifest in the person, there is nothing that is not influenced by it.

CHUANG TZU

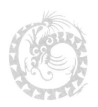

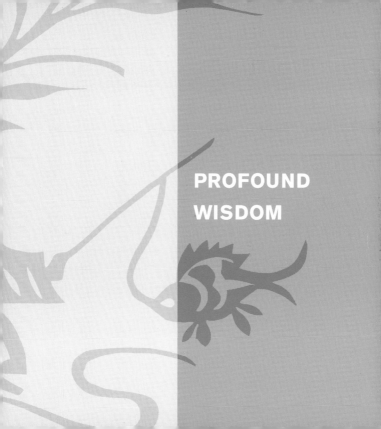

PROFOUND

WISDOM

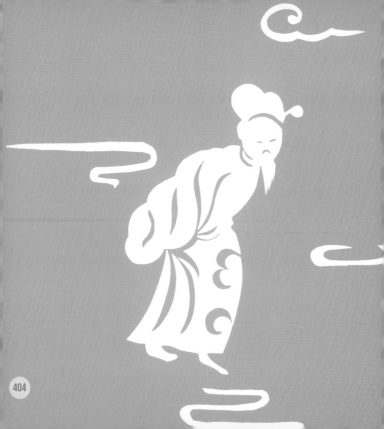

The ancients say that we must enjoy our life, free ourselves from worry, and take care of basic necessities. A good life is one in which we have our basic needs met, we have compassion, and we are able to enjoy ourselves.

Periodically, we should ask ourselves: Can we use compassion and kindness with strangers or people that we find strange? Can we extend ourselves to others, even when we don't know them? Can we offer what we have to those who have nothing, even when they are not our family or friends?

When we realize that whatever we have will be enough; when we are happy with whatever level of success we have attained; when we are willing to share our wealth and when we are not afraid of losing it; then we know that we have achieved true success!

By not being attached to loss or gain, by not feeling like a failure if we don't live up to our (or anyone else's) expectations, by not beating ourselves up over our perceived deficiencies, we can gift ourselves with the grace to let things unfold over time.

When we learn to be satisfied with what we have, then whatever else we are given will seem like treasure.

We must be open and empty in order to receive. If we are already full of plans, schemes, and doubts, how can we be fit to receive?

It is not enough to be born, to live, and then to die. What we do with our lives is what will live on after us. The people we touch, the other lives we influence, what good deeds we accomplish, what happiness we create—this will be the measure of our success.

The Tao gives birth to all things. So too, do we give birth to our own lives. Our personal good fortune depends on how much spiritual energy or merit we have accumulated. This is given freely by the Tao. All we need do is be open to it.

Good fortune follows those who give selflessly of what they have in order to receive what they need.

You've got to give what you've got, to get what you need.

Establishing your "bottom line," or what you need to survive in a healthy fashion, can give you a base line to work from.

Be willing to work for what you receive. Get-rich schemes seldom work. Trying to become prosperous through gambling seldom pays off.

In ancient times people did not have to plow and till the fields, because the seeds of grass and the fruit of the trees were enough for people to eat. They did not have to weave, because the skins of wild animals provided clothing. No one had to struggle to keep himself provided for.

At that time people were few and there was an abundance of everything, and so people did not quarrel. Therefore, there were no rich rewards offered or severe punishments doled out because the people, of themselves, were orderly.

Nowadays no one regards five sons as a large number and those sons each have five sons of their own and so by the time a man is a grandfather he has twenty-five grandchildren. And so the number of people has greatly increased, goods have grown scarce, and now people have to struggle and slave every day to make their living. Because of this, people have fallen to quarreling and, even though rewards are doubled and punishments are more severe, the people cannot be prevented from being disorderly.

HAN FEI TZU

In our modern, fast-moving society, restraint is almost a dirty word. Most people want whatever they want whenever they want it, regardless of the destructive influence it may have on them, the planet, or society as a whole.

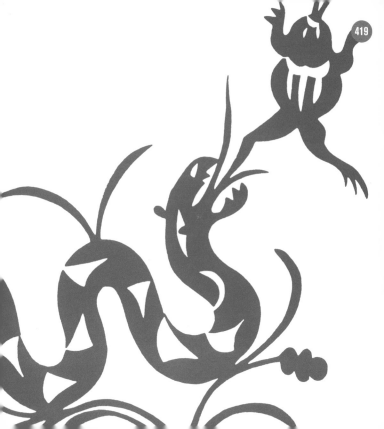

It is only in putting our faith, our resources, our resolve, our ambition, our destiny in the eternal that we have any hope of surviving beyond death.

People are often defeated

Just as they are on the verge of success.

If you are as careful at the end of an endeavor

As you are at the beginning,

You cannot fail.

LAO TZU

It is in paying attention to the details, as well as the greater vision, that we will be successful. By keeping things in perspective along the way we will be less likely to lose our place.

We must always keep in mind that we can lose everything we have in a moment. If we can remember that and still be able to enjoy our success we will have reached a high level of cultivation.

By simplifying one's activities, one's emotions, one's mind, and one's spirit, one becomes united with the very essence of the universe. One conducts oneself exactly as a natural being. Then the universe responds not to man's manipulative mind but to his pure spirit.

HUA CHING NI

By taking time to connect with our true nature, we can act in a spiritually responsible manner. It takes a deep understanding of our emotional, psychological, and energetic self before we can claim any sort of self-knowledge. This is where meditation or deep self-reflection comes in.

. . . if we do not succeed when others with the same abilities did; it feels good to find an excuse to get depressed and think that we are treated unfairly. However, if we can break free from this mode of thought and acknowledge that there are some things we simply cannot control, then there will be less disappointment, frustration and anger, and dissatisfaction in our lives.

EVA WONG

Often extremely successful people are so driven to attain success that, once they reach it, they can no longer enjoy it. Learn to enjoy what you have now and you will enjoy whatever else you attain that much more.

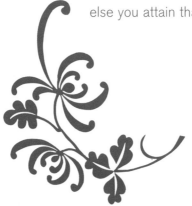

When dealing with movement or change,
the attitude which should be utilized is that
of the phase of Earth. Its force connotes
calmness, keeping to the root,
perceptiveness, maintain balance, and not
seeking extremes.

HUA CHING NI

Once there was a man named Ho, who, having found an uncut piece of jade in the Ch'u Mountains, brought it to the court and presented it to King Li. The king had his royal jeweler examine it, who, after a brief glance at it, announced it worthless. The king was angry, thinking that Ho was trying to deceive him and so ordered his left foot cut off as punishment.

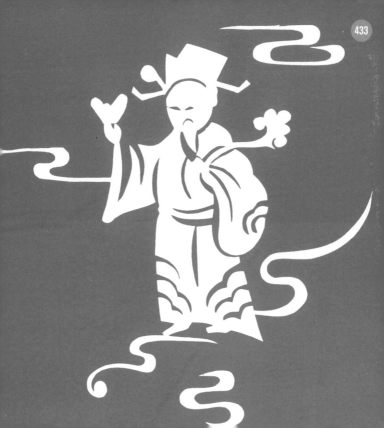

Years later King Li passed away and King Wu ascended to the throne. Ho presented his stone to the court once again, and once again the aged jeweler announced it a mere stone. The king thought that Ho was once again trying to deceive the throne and so ordered his right foot cut off.

Ho, clasping his stone to his chest, dragged himself to the foot of Ch'u mountain and wept piteously for three days and three nights. It is said that when all his tears were cried out he wept blood.

When the king heard about this he sent a servant to Ho who questioned him. "Many people have had this sort of punishment," the servant said to him. "Why do you weep so piteously over it?"

"I am not grieving over my lost feet," answered Ho. "I grieve because a precious jewel is called a mere stone and a man of integrity is called a deceiver."

When the king heard this he ordered the jeweler to cut and polish the stone, and when he did a precious jewel emerged.

HAN FEI TZU

Often our own talents can be hidden or overlooked. It may take some digging and some exploration to discover just what they are.

What is obvious is not always what is truly precious. If we take the time to look deeper into a situation or opportunity, what at first may seem worthless can become valuable.

Take time to explore just what it is that interests you. A life spent working at a job that you are unsuited for will only produce misery and regrets.

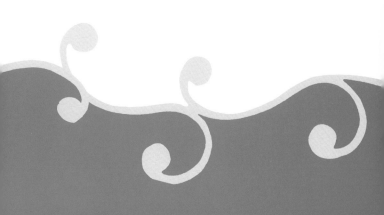

Most people never have the time or the opportunity to discover their own innate abilities. Instead they are shunted off into a career or job where they may have no interest and may spend their entire lives in boredom, frustration, and even depression.

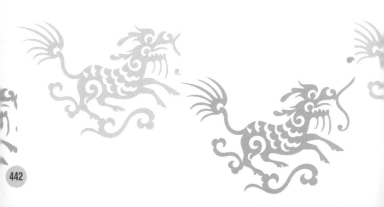

Ask yourself what it is that you are seeking from prosperity and how you can become clearer about your objectives.

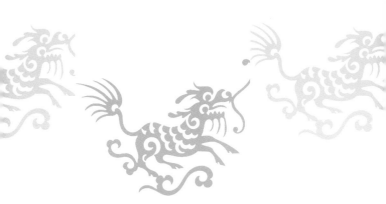

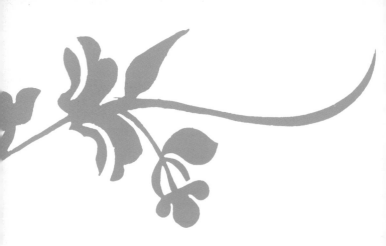

It is important to remember that when we do our own personal cultivation we are also affecting everyone around us—everyone that we have dealings with—emotionally, politically, businesswise, or interpersonally.

When we are not operating from a
sense of fear or negativity, we can
feel safe in our own natural being.

If I call you good, I am not speaking of your benevolence or righteousness. Goodness is simply one who possesses the qualities of Tao. If I say they are good, I am not speaking of what people call benevolence and righteousness, but simply of allowing the nature with which you have been endowed to have its free course. If I call you a good listener, I do not mean that you listen to anything other than your true self. If I pronounce you as being of clear vision, I do not mean to say that you see anything other than your own true self.

CHUANG TZU

Taoists believe that everyone is essentially good. It is only when their essential, natural goodness is distorted, stunted, or suppressed that they become something else.

448

The greatest happiness is achieved though a
higher understanding of the nature of things. For
the full development of oneself, one needs to
express one's innate ability.

VICTOR H. MAIR

What other people call goodness and righteousness may have nothing to do with natural virtue. Real virtue must come from the inside, not from what society calls goodness.

Be the kind of person that other people turn to when they have problems. You may not be able to solve everyone's problems, but you can, at least, give them some hope.

It is easy to be compassionate to those who seem inferior to you. It is easy to be compassionate to those who obviously need compassion and who return compassion to you. It is not so easy to be compassionate to those who are themselves uncompassionate but who need it so much more.

Through compassion we can learn to be soft. When we are soft, we can overcome the hardest thing in the world. Thus we can be valorous.

WANG AN SHIH

Because it is empty, the sage's
mind can receive.

Because it is still, it can respond.

The true sage does not make a show of him or herself. They do not advertise themselves as masters in glossy magazines, or charge exorbitant amounts for sharing their wisdom, or seduce their students with promises of personal energy transmission.

HUI TSANG

People who are always so concerned with following the rules, who never do anything that society might consider inappropriate, who are always influenced by what others might think of them—these people will never enjoy the wild freedom of being naturally and virtuously free.

If we content ourselves with the trimming of the branches and don't see to the roots, we may look fine on the outside, but will be rotten on the inside.

You must first win their hearts before you can command others.

WANG CHEN

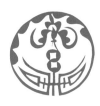

Solala Towler is a musican, poet, and teacher. He is editor of *The Empty Vessel, A Journal of Contemporary Taoism*, a magazine with an international subscription and distribution base (www.abodetao.com). He is also author of *A Gathering of Cranes: Bringing the Tao to the West* and *Embarking On the Way: A Guide to Western Taoism*. He is an instructor of Taoist meditation and of several styles of *chi gong*. He has taught classes and seminars all over the U.S. and abroad and is currently President of the National Qigong Association o USA.

Solala leads yearly tours to China to study *chi gong*, and visit Taoist temples and sacred mountains. You can email him at solala@abodetao.com or call (001)-541-345-8854.

First published by MQ Publications Limited
12 The Ivories, 6–8 Northhampton St., London, N1 2HY

Copyright © MQ Publications Limited 2002
Text © Solala Towler 2002
Design: Axis Design Editions

All materials quoted from the works of Hua Ching Ni are reprinted, with
permission, by SevenStar Communications., 13315 W. Washington Blvd.,
Ste. 200, Los Angeles, CA 90066

Library of Congress Cataloging-in-Publication Data
Towler, Solala
    Tao paths to good fortune/Solala Towler
        p. cm.
    ISBN: 0–7407–2295–6
    1. Fortune. 2. Tao. I. Title.

    BJ1611.2 T59 2002
    299.5144–dc21   2001046433

Printed and bound in China

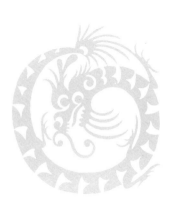

Bibliography

Blofeld, John. *Introduction to the Inner Structure of the I Ching* by Lama Anagarika Givinda. Wheelright Press, 1981.

Brown, Simon. *Practical Feng Shui*. London: Ward Lock, 1997.

Chuen, Master *Lam Kam*. *Feng Shui Handbook*. New York: Henry Holt, 1996.

Collins, Terah Kathryn. *The Western Guide to Feng Shui*. Carlsbad, Calif.: Hay House, Inc., 1996.

Cooper, J.C. *Taoism: The Way of the Mystic* Wellingborough, Northamptonshire: The Aquarian Press, 1972.

Eitel, Ernest J. with John Mitchell. *Feng-Shui: The Science of Sacred Landscape in Old China*. London: Synergetic Press, 1984.

Fischer-Schreiber, Ingrid. *The Shambhala Dictionary of Taoism*. Boston: Shambhala, 1996.

Graham, A.C., trans. *The Book of Lieh-tzu: A Classic of Tao*. New York: Columbia University Press, 1960.

Hamill, Sam and J.P. Seaton, trans. *The Essential Chuang Tzu*. Boston: Shambhala, 1998.

Knapp, Ronald G. China's *Vernacular Architecture: House Form and Culture*. Honolulu: University of Hawaii Press, 1989.

Levitt, Susan. *Taoist Feng Shui*. Rochester, VA: Destiny Books, 2000.

Mair, Victor H., trans.*Wandering on the Way: Early Taoist Tales and Parables of Chuang Tzu*. New York: Bantam, 1994.

Ming-Dao, Deng. 365 *Tao: Daily Meditations*. San Francisco: HarperSanFrancisco, 1992.

Ming-Dao, Deng. *Everyday Dao: Living with Balance and Harmony*. San Francisco: HarperSanFrancisco, 1996.

Ni, Hua-Ching. *The Book of Changes and The Unchanging Truth*. Los Angeles: The Shrine of the Eternal Breath of Tao and College of Tao and Traditional Chinese Healing, 1983.

Ni, Hua-Ching. *Life and Teaching of Two Immortals, Vol. II: Chen Tuan*. Santa Monica: Seven Star, 1993.

Ni, Hua-Ching. *Tao: The Subtle Universal Law and the Intergral Way of Life*. Los Angeles: College of Tao and Traditional Chinese Healing, 1979.

Richter, Gregory C. *The Gate of All Marvelous Things*. Red Mansions Publishing, 1998.

Rossbach, Sarah. *Interior Design with Feng Shui*. New York: E.P. Dutton, 1987.

Waltham, Clae. *Chuang Tzu: Genius of the Absurd*. New York: Ace Books, 1971.

Watson, Burton, trans. *Han Fei Tzu: Basic Writings*. New York: Columbia University Press, 1964.

Wong, Eva. *Feng-Shui: The American Wisdom of Harmonious Living for Modern Times*. Boston: Shambhala, 1996.

Wong, Eva. *Lieh-tzu: A Taoist Guide to Practical Living*. New York: Ace Books, 1971.

Xin, Yan. *Secrets and Benefits of Internal Qigong Cultivation*. Malvern, PA: Amber Leaf Press, 1997.

Yu-lan, Fung, trans. by Derek Bodde. *A History of Chinese Philosophy: Vol. II*. Princeton: Princeton University Press, 1953.